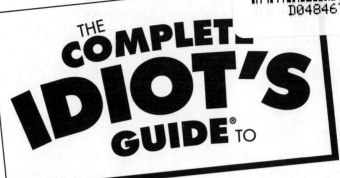

THE
COMPLETE
IDIOT'S
GUIDE® TO

Medical Care for the Uninsured

by Mark L. Friedman, M.D., and Donna Raskin

ALPHA

A member of Penguin Group (USA) Inc.

This book is dedicated to the doctors, nurses, and other providers who care for, and care about, the uninsured. It is especially dedicated to emergency physicians who make a career of treating all patients, regardless of their ability to pay. MF

ALPHA BOOKS

Published by the Penguin Group

Penguin Group (USA) Inc., 375 Hudson Street, New York, New York 10014, USA

Penguin Group (Canada), 90 Eglinton Avenue East, Suite 700, Toronto, Ontario M4P 2Y3, Canada (a division of Pearson Penguin Canada Inc.)

Penguin Books Ltd., 80 Strand, London WC2R 0RL, England

Penguin Ireland, 25 St. Stephen's Green, Dublin 2, Ireland (a division of Penguin Books Ltd.)

Penguin Group (Australia), 250 Camberwell Road, Camberwell, Victoria 3124, Australia (a division of Pearson Australia Group Pty. Ltd.)

Penguin Books India Pvt. Ltd., 11 Community Centre, Panchsheel Park, New Delhi—110 017, India

Penguin Group (NZ), 67 Apollo Drive, Rosedale, North Shore, Auckland 1311, New Zealand (a division of Pearson New Zealand Ltd.)

Penguin Books (South Africa) (Pty.) Ltd., 24 Sturdee Avenue, Rosebank, Johannesburg 2196, South Africa

Penguin Books Ltd., Registered Offices: 80 Strand, London WC2R 0RL, England

International Standard Book Number: 978-1-59257-734-7
Library of Congress Catalog Card Number: 2007939744

10 09 08   8 7 6 5 4 3 2 1

Interpretation of the printing code: The rightmost number of the first series of numbers is the year of the book's printing; the rightmost number of the second series of numbers is the number of the book's printing. For example, a printing code of 08-1 shows that the first printing occurred in 2008.

Printed in the United States of America

Note: This publication contains the opinions and ideas of its authors. It is intended to provide helpful and informative material on the subject matter covered. It is sold with the understanding that the authors and publisher are not engaged in rendering professional services in the book. If the reader requires personal assistance or advice, a competent professional should be consulted.

The authors and publisher specifically disclaim any responsibility for any liability, loss, or risk, personal or otherwise, which is incurred as a consequence, directly or indirectly, of the use and application of any of the contents of this book.

Most Alpha books are available at special quantity discounts for bulk purchases for sales promotions, premiums, fund-raising, or educational use. Special books, or book excerpts, can also be created to fit specific needs.

For details, write: Special Markets, Alpha Books, 375 Hudson Street, New York, NY 10014.

Publisher: *Marie Butler-Knight*
Editorial Director: *Mike Sanders*
Senior Managing Editor: *Billy Fields*
Acquisitions Editor: *Tom Stevens*
Development Editor: *Michael Thomas*
Production Editor: *Megan Douglass*

Copy Editor: *Nancy Wagner*
Cover Designer: *Bill Thomas*
Book Designer: *Trina Wurst*
Indexer: *Heather McNeill*
Layout: *Brian Massey*
Proofreader: *Mary Hunt*

Contents at a Glance

Contents

Introduction

Today in the United States the quality of one's health depends not only on his family history and how well he takes care of himself but also on whether or not he has insurance. In general, Americans without insurance don't go to the doctor for preventive care, which means that if they have an illness, they are diagnosed when their disease is at a more advanced stage, and, finally, once diagnosed, the uninsured receive less care and die more often and sooner than people with insurance. In fact, throughout every stage of health and disease, no matter what the type of care, including general health, mental health, dental health, and specific diseases, Americans without insurance fare worse than those with insurance, according to the National Coalition on Health Care, an organization whose honorary co-chairs are former Presidents George Bush and Jimmy Carter.

It was certainly not always true that insurance was equal to health care in America, but just as medical breakthroughs have allowed us to live longer and better, the cost of health care has risen precipitously while, at the same time, the American economy has shifted from a manufacturing-based economy to a service economy. These changes in the job market as well as the population's general health and more advanced medical care have created a perfect storm of cost and need and availability, which has negatively affected the health-care industry (but certainly not the health insurance industry, which has seen rising profits during this transition).

Since the mid-1950s most Americans have received health insurance through their employers as a benefit counted above and beyond their salary. But since about the year 2000, employment is no longer a guarantee of health insurance coverage. There are a number of reasons for this change:

◆ The move from manufacturing to service has reduced how many businesses offer insurance to employees.

◆ More companies use part-time and contract or consultant workers who are not eligible for health insurance. In fact, by law, companies do not have to offer insurance to these workers because they aren't technically employees.

- Because health insurance premiums are so expensive, small employers often can't afford to offer health benefits to their employees.

- Medium and large-size companies that do offer health insurance now have to ask their employees to contribute more money toward their coverage. Because these premiums are so expensive, more Americans simply go without insurance rather than paying the premium.

Because of these circumstances, about 47 million Americans (16 percent of the population) did not have health insurance in 2005. This means the number of uninsured people rose by 1.3 million between 2004 and 2005 and has increased by almost 7 million people since 2000.

Because of these increased costs, over 8 in 10 uninsured people come from working families of middle-income status. In fact, nearly 40 percent of the uninsured (this number includes children and other dependents) live in households that earn $50,000 or more. Think about it: if a family of four has an income of $50,000 a year (or $961 a week before taxes) and their insurance costs average $11,000 a year (or $211 a week), that expense reflects almost 30 percent of an untaxed income. That cost would have to fight its way into a budget that includes a mortgage or rent, food, clothing, and education, not to mention incidentals.

But of course, the insurance catastrophe is not just affecting the poor and the working. In 2003, 11.2 percent of all children in the United States were uninsured. This number increased by nearly 400,000 in 2005. Nearly 50 percent of uninsured children did not receive a checkup in 2003, almost twice the rate (26 percent) for insured children.

But here's the most painful irony: the cost of insurance doesn't have to reflect the ability of the American health-care system to deliver good health care. American doctors and hospitals are among the best in the world. If you have a life-threatening disease, such as cancer, you could benefit from groundbreaking research and state-of-the-art treatment. If you see a primary care physician regularly, you have a doctor who can provide you with tests and exams that will detect almost all problems in the early stages.

Nevertheless, in 2000, the World Health Organization rated the United States thirty-seventh in health-care systems around the world. That's because although Americans spend $5,267 per capita on health care (two and half times the world medium), the extra spending goes toward paperwork, not health care.

In the end, Americans have fewer doctors per capita than other industrialized countries, go to the doctor fewer times each year, go to the hospital less, and, because of all these things, are also less happy with our doctors and medical care system. Even worse, we die sooner than those who live in other industrialized countries. And the problems exist throughout the lifespan; our children get fewer immunizations and have a higher infant mortality.

Of course, not having insurance in America doesn't mean you don't get any health care. People without insurance often try to pay for their own health care or qualify for government insurance. Sometimes uninsured patients rely on physicians, clinics, and hospitals to take them on as patients without asking for pay. Numerous programs try to help the uninsured see doctors, get exams and tests, and get the health care insured patients receive.

To our way of thinking, good health care means you like your doctor, can afford appropriate preventative tests and examinations, and feel as if you would be well cared for if you got sick or had a medical emergency. Is it possible for everyone in America to get good health care, regardless of insurance?

Free Your Mind and Your Health Will Follow

Have you ever heard the word paradigm? It's a great word, although its not commonly used. It means framework or a model or pattern for how you create a way of thinking. So, let's say you are a parent and you're thinking about how you are going to spend your day. Because of your children, your paradigm for your planning necessarily includes the needs of your kids. But, if you're single, your paradigm wouldn't include worrying about children. A parent and a single person have different paradigms when it comes to time organization.

Well, when it comes to health care, many Americans think insurance, not health care. In other words, Americans have been trained to think that how healthy we are and the kind of medical care we receive is equal to how good our insurance is. And, in fact, as we write this book, they're right. As we said, Americans without insurance don't get the health care that those with insurance do.

But, we hope this book will help you live healthfully no matter what your insurance situation. Although it's easier to find a doctor and pay her, or go to a hospital and pay for services with insurance, you don't necessarily need insurance to find a doctor or to get medical tests or have surgery. There are ways to get the care you need without insurance. And we're here to help you do that.

In some cases, the advice we give you will involve little or no cost. In others, you can expect to pay for the care you receive. You need to realize that no one who receives regular health care gets it for free. People in other countries who have access to complete health care insurance pay for the services they receive through taxes and frequently supplement the cost with other payments.

The bottom line is this: some portion of your income (assuming you have one) will have to go toward health care. The question is: what portion will that be and how do you want to spend that money?

In this book you will learn about all of your health-care options so that you can make informed decisions for your body, mind, spirit—and wallet.

What's in This Book

This book is divided into three parts.

Part 1, "Getting Coverage No Matter What Your Situation," provides an overview of the healthcare situation in America today and explains that you may have access to insurance coverage you didn't know about. It also features a chapter on creating your own insurance plan.

In **Part 2, "Getting Care on an Ongoing Basis,"** we cover the basics of getting ongoing care, with special chapters focusing on women, children, and those aged 50–65. You'll also find chapters on mental health care, dental and vision care, and elective surgery.

Part 3, "When You Need Care Now," focuses on emergencies and determining when you should and shouldn't go to an emergency room. This part also addresses the problems of fighting denied claims and working out your own payment plan.

Extras

Throughout the book, you'll see sidebars that contain important information.

For Your Health

These sidebars feature helpful tips.

Code Red

These boxes contain warnings you'll need to be aware of.

def•i•ni•tion

These sidebars define important terms.

Bet You Didn't Know

Here you'll find interesting facts and information.

Trademarks

All terms mentioned in this book that are known to be or are suspected of being trademarks or service marks have been appropriately capitalized. Alpha Books and Penguin Group (USA) Inc. cannot attest to the accuracy of this information. Use of a term in this book should not be regarded as affecting the validity of any trademark or service mark.

Part 1

Getting Coverage No Matter What Your Situation

Forty-seven million Americans do not have healthcare coverage, and you may be one of them. That doesn't mean you're without options, however. In Part 1, we take a thorough look at the healthcare situation in America, sort through the alphabet soup of insurance options (many of those who are uninsured do have access to insurance, and many with insurance don't fully understand their policies), and provide you with the basics for taking charge of your one-of-a-kind situation.

Chapter 1

Not Every Uninsured Person Is the Same

In This Chapter

- ◆ Coping with unemployment
- ◆ Living with a disability
- ◆ The truth about "free" health care for illegal immigrants
- ◆ Insuring a preexisting condition
- ◆ Getting health care for your employees

The statistic is alarming—47 million Americans are uninsured, but in this case, there is no safety in numbers. In fact, knowing that you aren't alone probably doesn't make you feel any better. The truth is, this number is so overwhelming and upsetting that it probably makes you feel a little hopeless. After all, if 46.999999 million other Americans can't figure out how to get insurance—and perhaps medical attention—then how are you going to?

The reality is that you need health care, and even though you are one of many, your story is one-of-a-kind. To get better health care, you need to know how the specifics of your situation (maybe you are unemployed, have a disability, or are self-employed) will contribute to the decisions you make regarding your health care.

The Unemployed Uninsured

Most Americans get their health insurance as a *benefit* through their jobs, so job loss is frightening and threatening to Americans, not just because of income loss but also because of the fear of losing their health insurance.

def•i•ni•tion

A **benefit** is something an employer offers as an advantage above and beyond one's salary. Most companies, according to the Robert Wood Johnson Foundation, spend 41 cents for benefits (health care, vacation, life insurance, etc.) for every dollar on payroll. Nevertheless, very few employers pay all of the health-care costs for their employees. In fact, American employees paid an average annual amount of $3,481 in health insurance costs in 2003.

In fact, you probably know many people who keep their jobs because of their health insurance benefit. Let's consider Sarah, a factory worker in Michigan. Sarah went to school to be a massage therapist and has about five clients a week, above and beyond her full-time job at the factory. She knows she could easily get more clients, but her job provides a pretty good health insurance benefit. Sarah pays $250 a month toward her health insurance premium, but her insurance gives her medical, dental, and vision care. She went shopping for a comparable health insurance plan, but as far as she could tell, it would cost her about $1,300 a month to receive all of those benefits. Sarah doesn't like her job—she loves being a massage therapist—but in no way can she match the benefits of her company if she strikes out on her own.

So Sarah, and perhaps you, have a hard choice to make. Sometimes, you just can't stick with a job you hate. But at other times, you stay because the insurance is so important to you or someone in your family.

Unfortunately, of course, you may not always have a choice about keeping a job because of its good benefits. Circumstances may force you to leave a job, or maybe you must move away. Whatever the reason, few of us keep our jobs—good insurance or not—forever. A change from full-time to part-time work, self-employment, retirement, or divorce can also cut a person's link to employer-sponsored coverage.

If you had a job—or are about to leave a job—that had good health insurance (and by "good" we mean your premium was affordable and your coverage allowed you to get the medical care you needed and wanted), you will most likely be offered COBRA coverage when you leave your employer.

Bet You Didn't Know

How did employers become a source of health insurance? There was a nationwide wage freeze during World War II, so employers used pension plans, profit sharing, and health insurance plans to attract employees. This benefit became a standard expectation for most employees—and helped the insurance industry grow, too!

COBRA

COBRA stands for Consolidated Omnibus Budget Reconciliation Act, a law the United States Congress passed in 1985 which allows employees to continue their health insurance benefit for about 18 months after they leave their job, if there are 20 or more employees in the company. You can opt to get COBRA benefits no matter how you end up leaving your job unless you are guilty of gross misconduct, such as violence or drinking on the job. If you are disabled, you can often continue your health insurance benefits for up to 29 months.

If you qualify for COBRA benefits, your coverage will be identical to the coverage provided under the group health plan, but here's the kicker: COBRA is much more expensive than your traditional health insurance from your employer. In fact, you will have to pay the entire premium for coverage plus a small administrative fee.

Code Red

Only seven percent of unemployed people can afford to pay for COBRA. Premiums are typically $700 to $1,000 a month for family coverage.

In other words, you must pay the total cost of your health insurance, including what your employer paid as part of your benefits package. You have 60 days to accept COBRA coverage; if you do not accept the offer within 60 days, you lose all rights to benefits.

Bet You Didn't Know

If you change jobs and already have an illness or disease, such as diabetes or you are HIV+, your new company's health plan may have a "preexisting condition" clause. This means that you will not receive any benefits for the treatment of the medical conditions you had prior to getting your new insurance. You can use your COBRA benefits from your previous employer to cover your preexisting condition. Preexisting condition clauses usually expire after one year, and then you can receive full coverage.

COBRA benefits are also available to spouses and children of covered employees. You can also use COBRA for dental, vision, and prescription drug plans.

Unfortunately, COBRA benefits can be very expensive. In fact, the better your insurance and the larger your company, the more costly your insurance will be! But remember that COBRA is a choice. It may be less expensive, especially over the long run, for you to choose a different type of coverage.

Insurance as Part of Unemployment Benefits

If you are unemployed, COBRA is not your only option. For example, if you are eligible for unemployment benefits, you may also be eligible for health insurance. Depending on the state you live in, your financial status, and previous health insurance, you may be offered full coverage at no cost or some level of coverage with some of the cost handled by the state. Most state unemployment offices will explain this benefit to you when you apply. You can also see Appendix B for more information.

Code Red

The shock of losing your job is a big one, but don't let your health insurance go just because you're afraid. It's better to accept COBRA coverage and use it for a month or two than to not choose it and have no health insurance when you really need it.

You also have some other options. First, you may be able to get health insurance through a professional organization (see "Insurance for the Self-Employed" in this chapter). If you are a veteran or have a disability, there are government programs that will provide you with healthcare as well as insurance.

The point is, even if you are "unemployed," you might do better to think of yourself as a freelancer or some other category that often means you can get health insurance or medical care without using COBRA. So, don't assume that this is the only section of this book that can help you get health care. Instead, think of being unemployed as just one category in which you might be included—temporarily—and that may help you get insurance. You probably have other options if you need them, so keep reading.

Insurance for the Disabled

You might be surprised to learn that you don't get to decide for yourself whether you're disabled—other people determine that. And the guidelines regarding who is disabled are hard to understand.

To be eligible for disability insurance as well as social programs for disabled persons, you must document a variety of doctors' diagnoses as well as your work and financial history.

Bet You Didn't Know

Most employers provide disability insurance to their employees, which will replace a portion of your income if you can't work because of an injury or illness. Short-term disability provides an income for the early part of a disability, from two weeks to a few months. Then, long-term disability may kick in, which helps replace income for an extended period of time. If you have any type of insurance, call the insurance company to see if disability is included in your plan.

Medicaid provides medical care for certain individuals and families with low incomes and resources. This program, which became law in 1965, is jointly funded by federal and state governments, including the District of Columbia and U.S. Territories, and allows states to provide medical care to people who meet certain eligibility criteria.

Medicaid covers many groups of people, but even within these groups, a patient must meet certain requirements regarding age; condition, whether pregnant, disabled, blind, or aged; income and resources; and one's status as a U.S. citizen or a lawfully admitted immigrant. The rules for counting a person's income and resources vary between states and groups. Those who live in nursing homes and disabled children who live at home have special rules.

Code Red

Medicare and Medicaid are two entirely different programs. Medicare is a federal health insurance program for people over 65 and for those on Social Security disability who have met specific disability guidelines, such as those with irreversible kidney failure or Lou Gehrig's Disease (ALS). Medicaid, on the other hand, is an assistance program funded jointly by the federal government and individual states, which provides benefits to low-income citizens for long-term care due to illness. Both are part of the Social Services program.

Medicaid is a state-administered program, and each state sets its own guidelines subject to federal rules. States must cover certain services in order to receive federal funds, such as in- and outpatient hospital services, doctor visits, and long-term care services, such as nursing home care or community-based care, among others. Additional services are optional and are elected by states. For example, coverage of prescription drugs is an optional state benefit; however, every state and the District of Columbia provide prescription drug coverage to Medicaid enrollees.

To apply for Medicaid in your state, contact your local Medicaid office. For contact information, look in the blue pages of your phone book, probably under "Medical Assistance." Some states let you apply on the Internet, by telephone, or at locations in the community, such as community health centers. By contacting Medicaid directly, you can get state information.

Illegal Immigrants and Healthcare

The truth is, citizens are far more likely to have health insurance and get better health care than illegal immigrants. And the statistic is significant: 13 percent of native-born citizens lacked health insurance in 2005, while 43 percent of noncitizens did. And that statistic is clearly low since people who are in the country illegally don't eagerly answer survey questions. Nevertheless, no one is really sure how much the immigrant population affects the insurance industry. Each side of the issue has its own set of statistics, and those numbers are so wildly different that it is impossible to figure out the reality.

According to an August 2007 article in *The New England Journal of Medicine*,

> … although anti-immigrant sentiment is fueled by the belief that immigrants can obtain federal benefits, 1996 welfare-reform legislation greatly restricted immigrants' access to programs such as Medicaid, shifting most health-care responsibility to state and local governments. The law requires that immigrants wait 5 years after obtaining lawful permanent residency (a "green card") to apply for federal benefits. In response, some states and localities—for instance, Illinois, New York, the District of Columbia, and certain California counties—have used their own funds to expand health insurance coverage even for undocumented immigrant children and pregnant women with low incomes. Other states, however, such as Arizona, Colorado, Georgia, and Virginia, have passed laws making it even more difficult for noncitizens to gain access to health services.

Whether or not they have health insurance, immigrants overall have much lower per capita health-care expenditures than native-born Americans, and recent analyses indicate that they contribute more to the economy in taxes than they receive in public benefits. In a study from the RAND Corporation, researchers estimated that undocumented adult immigrants, who make up about 3.2 percent of the population, account for only about 1.5 percent of U.S. medical costs.

Now, if a person—any person—shows up at an emergency room, the clerk at the desk will ask the nature of the emergency, as well as for insurance information. If the patient has a true emergency (a heart attack, for example), the doctor will not refuse to care for the patient based on immigration or insurance status.

Bet You Didn't Know

Remember, emergency treatment isn't "free" for anyone. Everyone is billed and expected to pay for treatment. Some hospitals and doctors are willing to write off all or part of a bill based on a person's circumstances, but remember that while emergency care is a "right," guaranteed by the Emergency Medical Treatment and Active Labor Act (EMTALA), it nevertheless comes with a "responsibility," i.e., payment for services.

But emergency care doesn't continue indefinitely. Once a person has stabilized, then treatment is no longer "guaranteed." Other providers of care, such as walk-in clinics and private doctors, expect payment. Some physicians do accept charity cases without asking for the immigration status of any person, while others will ask. All physicians, except emergency physicians, have the right to decide who they treat and for what amount of money. They also have the right to decide which insurance plans to accept or not, including Medicare, Medicaid, and other government programs.

Covering Preexisting Medical Conditions

Under the law, most of which went into effect on July 1, 1997, a *preexisting condition* will be covered without a waiting period when you join a new group plan if you have been insured the previous 12 months. This means that if you remain insured for 12 months or more, you will be able to go from one job to another, and your preexisting condition will be covered—without additional waiting periods—even if you have a chronic illness. For this reason it is important to avoid any gaps in coverage by using the COBRA insurance option if necessary between jobs.

def•i•ni•tion

A **preexisting condition** is a medical condition for which a person has been diagnosed or treated before joining a new plan. In the past, health care given for a preexisting condition often was not covered for someone who joined a new plan until after a waiting period.

If you have a preexisting condition and have not been insured the previous 12 months before joining a new plan, the longest you will have to wait before you are covered for that condition is 12 months.

For Your Health _____

Preexisting conditions aren't always illnesses. We know a woman who switched jobs a few years ago, and in between the two, she became pregnant—and her new employer's plan wouldn't cover her. So, always make sure you think ahead (if possible!) when you are changing jobs to make sure you don't lose coverage. Fortunately, the Health Insurance Portability and Accountability Act (HIPAA) says that pregnancy can no longer be classified as a preexisting condition.

However, HIPAA changes the rules. If you have had coverage for the preceding 12 months in a group plan (18 months in an individual plan), then your new employer must waive any preexisting limits to coverage. Be careful with this rule, though. If you go through two months without coverage (such as if you don't sign on to COBRA), then you may not qualify since your coverage had what is called a "significant break."

You can also ask the insurance company if it's possible to get a "rider" on the policy that excludes the preexisting condition. A rider means the insurance won't pay for care related to this specific condition but will pay for other care. You have to be careful about this, though, as many insurance companies will then question the appearance of new illnesses and claims related to them. On the other hand, if your condition isn't very serious and you mostly just need preventative care, to get the insurance with the rider might be financially worthwhile.

Insurance for the Self-Employed

In some ways it would help if everyone reading this book thought of himself as being "self-employed" because a person who is his own boss must accept a primary reality about healthcare: he is in charge of his insurance and medical care.

If you are self-employed, you can't expect your employer to pay health insurance as a benefit and, at the same time, you have to make a decision about whether or not you need insurance. And, if you do need insurance, you then have to decide what type of coverage you need and want to pay for.

As we've said, there is a difference between health insurance and health care, so the first thing you need to ask yourself is, "What kind of health care do I need?" We address this question in Chapter 4, but you need to keep some considerations in mind if you are self-employed.

First, workers of almost all kinds, including writers and artists, can join unions or organizations composed of workers like themselves, most of which offer health insurance plans to their members. So, if you're a computer consultant or a graphic designer, look for these types of organizations and find out about the programs they offer. You can usually choose from different plans that will fulfill your needs.

Of course, as a private contractor, you need to pay your insurance premiums yourself, but you can work with an accountant to find out how to do this in the most advantageous way. Many health-care costs are tax-deductible, but only if you're earning more than the cost of the health care (in other words, if you're a starving artist, you may not be able to do this).

As a self-employed person, you need to work out your health insurance payments as part of your financial budget.

If You're Employed but Have Special Insurance Issues

Perhaps you are someone who has a job you love. And, lucky you, your employer offers health insurance as a benefit. Perhaps, like someone we know, you are a preschool teacher, a worthy job, of course, but one that doesn't pay a great deal. Meanwhile, your husband is a chef at a restaurant that is only open during the summer, so his employer is not required to offer a health insurance benefit.

The preschool teacher, a friend of ours, makes about $20,000 per year while her husband earns about $40,000. Preschools aren't a high margin business (i.e., there isn't a lot of profit for the owner), so a teacher pays close to 50 percent of her insurance premium. And what is the result? After taxes and insurance, this dedicated teacher brings home $100 every week. So why does she keep her job? Well, besides loving it, she is essentially working for her insurance because not having a salary and having to pay 100 percent of her premium is certainly more costly than the current situation.

Most of the uninsured individuals in the United States are working but earn less than 200 percent of the poverty level, according to the Kaiser Commission on Medicaid and the Uninsured. Nevertheless, these people work.

> **Code Red**
>
> Part-time workers make up only 19 percent of the population but are 28 percent of the uninsured.

In 2006, employer health insurance premiums increased by 7.7 percent, which is two times the rate of inflation. The annual premium for an employer health plan covering a family of four averaged nearly $11,500. The annual premium for individual coverage averaged over $4,200.

Employers are well aware of this situation, too. In fact, in many cases, employers might want employees who don't earn high wages to drop out of health coverage all together, as this reduces the cost to the employer.

> **Bet You Didn't Know**
>
> During the second world war, when medical benefits were first granted to employees, the general population was relatively young and workers had to pass a physical to get benefits. So, medical benefits cost about ½ of 1 percent of payroll. Now, for many companies the medical cost is well above 5 percent of payroll.

This strategy is working, too, because fewer and fewer employees are accepting their employer's offer of insurance. In fact, only about 80 percent of workers accept health insurance coverage. Even state workers are turning down the offer of insurance, mostly because of its expense.

Nevertheless, many employers are still expected to pay the great majority of the insurance premium, so if it's offered to you, it might be worth getting. Of course, you can also look into purchasing your own health insurance policy through a union or organization or try to find cost effective private insurance.

Sometimes, buying your own insurance plan is less expensive than sticking with an employer's, but it may still be expensive.

Insurance and the Small Business Owner

If you have a small company, which employs at least two but no more than fifty people, *small business* health insurance can benefit both you and your employees alike. When you choose a group plan, you can save on personal health-care costs, increase tax deductions, and boost job satisfaction within your company.

Group Health Insurance

Besides providing medical care for yourself and your employees, a small business health insurance plan helps spread the financial risk among all the members, which usually means lower premiums and more extensive coverage for everyone in your company. This is a clear win-win situation. In fact, small companies are combined into "risk pools" consisting of many small employers. Doing this actually helps to spread the risk over thousands of people rather than just dozens.

def•i•ni•tion

What constitutes a **Small Business**? According to the U.S. Small Business Administration (SBA), it depends on the industry. The designation can be based on a company's average annual receipts or on the company's average number of workers However, HIPAA defines a small business as one with 2 to 50 employees. Most states use the definition set by HIPAA, although some states include groups of one in their definition (see state by state regulations in Chapter 2 for more details).

Group health insurance has tax advantages too. Employer contributions to a small business health insurance plan are generally 100 percent tax deductible, and employees will save on their payroll taxes.

Certain other groups, such as nonprofit organizations, are also generally eligible for group health insurance as long as they can demonstrate that they have two or more full-time taxable employees.

A small business health insurance plan provides coverage for its members with rates calculated on a kind of bulk rate for the group. Employees may be able to add their own policy riders and have additional coverage to customize the policy to meet their specific needs, such as adding or subtracting optical or family care, but the basic policy format will remain the same for the whole group.

Likewise, though small business health insurance comes in a variety of shapes and sizes (e.g., fee-for-service, HMO, PPO, POS, all of which we explain in-depth in Chapter 2), the format that you choose for the company will apply to all the group members. It is possible to purchase a group indemnity policy, but the managed care plans are more affordable for every pay scale and, therefore, are much more common.

For a variety of reasons, health insurance premiums are calculated differently both from state to state and from company to company. The cost of a group health insurance plan is based on the characteristics of each individual member of the group, including, but of course not limited to, age, health status, occupational hazard, business and/or residential location, and lifestyle habits, including smoking and weight.

> **Bet You Didn't Know**
>
> Healthcare costs are thought to be one of the reasons for the outsourcing boom. Very few large companies can keep the insurance system the way it is unless they move their production offshore where the cost of health insurance is supported by tax on citizens.

Employees of businesses that offer group health insurance are not compelled to join the plan, but the group must maintain a minimum number of insured (as few as two people, depending on the policy) to guarantee coverage. Remember, though, that an individual purchasing the same type and amount of coverage will pay less in a group than if he purchased it individually.

No insurance company in any state can refuse to sell a group small group health insurance provided they offer coverage to other small groups and the group meets the state's minimum requirements concerning the type of organization they are insuring and the number of members in that group. Find out about the rules and protections applicable to small group insurance in your state by reading the information in Chapter 2.

The bottom line is no more or less than this: group health insurance is less expensive than a bunch of individual policies. This is a fact. However, it still is not cheap. No health care in America is.

The employer will be required to pay some percentage of an employee's individual premium, which is often 25 percent or 50 percent, depending, again, on the state's laws and the insurance company. Also if the employee wants to extend coverage to a spouse or dependant, the employer may choose to pay a percentage of that cost but is not required to do so. You will likely have several policy and payment options from which to choose.

Bet You Didn't Know

If you and your spouse both get health insurance at work, it may make more financial sense for you to be covered with different policies. Look at the options you both have that will best cover you and any children you have for the least amount of money. Don't assume that one spouse should automatically carry the whole family. And if you don't accept insurance from one employer, find out if you can be compensated in some way for the money you are saving your employer.

To get an accurate quote on a small business health insurance policy, you need reliable information about both the type of coverage you seek and the vital statistics of the group members who want to be insured, including the number of dependants they would like to include.

Not having all this information on hand is not a problem as you will be asked only for estimates to shop for quotes. No price is set in stone until you sign your name to paper; everything is an estimate until then. Just keep in mind the more accurate the information you provide, the more accurate the quote you receive.

In the long run, you will probably save money if you hire a benefits consultant in order to best choose among the many types of health plans.

Group health insurance is cheaper than individual policies because they allow insurers to spread the costs of treating everyone across all policyholders. So while an older member might need extra medical care, a younger one might rarely use the system. This makes it a little cheaper for the older, unhealthier group and a little more expensive for their younger counterparts.

HSAs

Depending on the type of business you own and the health and ages of your employees, you might consider encouraging your employees to open Health Savings Accounts in addition to your health-care plan. This program became an option recently, as part of the Health Opportunity Patient Empowerment Act of 2006.

Health Savings Accounts (HSA) provide employees with a savings account that earns interest and is tax-free when the money is used for medical charges. These accounts are perfect for younger employees who don't use medical care as often as older employees, so the money is able to grow with interest. HSAs are good investments for small business owners because when the employee leaves her job and the company, the money stays with the employer.

HSA accounts are typically set up alongside high deductible policies. This allows access to lower premiums and offers the potential of more control over a business's health-care dollar. That's because the employee makes more front end payments for physical exams, office visits, simple lab tests, etc., while the employer provides catastrophic coverage for claims an individual cannot afford to bear, such as hospital bills, surgeries, and long-term illness (see Chapter 3).

The Least You Need to Know

◆ Every situation has its own set of circumstances, but everyone needs to take charge of his healthcare and health insurance.

◆ Research your options and keep records of the information you receive from doctors, insurance companies, and everyone else involved in your care.

◆ Call your state's Medicaid office to see if you are covered through this federal program. Each state has its own set of rules and regulations.

◆ If you become unemployed, sign up for COBRA insurance so that you don't lose that choice, but do more research on other insurance to see if less expensive alternatives are available to you.

◆ If you own a business and want to insure yourself and your employees, hire a benefits consultant who can navigate the web of insurance options for you.

2

Sorting Through Your Insurance Options

In This Chapter

- ◆ Indemnity, PPO, HMO, and POS plans
- ◆ The difference between public and private health plans
- ◆ State by state health insurance regulations
- ◆ The answer to expensive medication or regular care
- ◆ No need to see a doctor, but maybe an emergency

Why are we discussing insurance options in a guide for the uninsured? Because many of those who are currently uninsured do in fact have access to insurance and many people with insurance do not fully understand their policies or how to make the most cost-effective insurance choices. In order to have access to the best health care it is almost always advisable to have some kind of health insurance if it is available to you.

In 2006, Michael went back to graduate school after working 20 years for large companies all around the United States. At each job he had had great health benefits at very little cost to him.

So, going back to school full-time didn't only mean forgoing a steady income but also giving up health insurance. He was stunned when a) his graduate school insisted that he had to purchase health insurance through them at a cost of $2,000 annually (which wouldn't cover his wife) and b) he found out he and his family were eligible for free health insurance through the state and he could choose between an HMO (Health Maintenance Organization) plan and a PPO (Preferred Provider Organization) plan (we explain both plans in a minute).

In other words, losing employer-sponsored health insurance doesn't mean that you aren't eligible for any health insurance. As we said in Chapter 1, you are eligible for COBRA, but you also have other options. You will see lots of ideas and suggestions for how you can get the health care you need without insurance in Part 2 of the book. But it is true that insurance will help you get better health care and that you will have to pay for health care whether you pay a doctor straight out of your pocket or you pay an insurance premium. Certainly, charity care and government assistance is an option for some (and we'll show you how to find out if it is right for you), but it is not necessarily the right choice for every person.

For Your Health

Choose a physician because she spends time listening to you and has experience with the health issues that worry you. Don't equate her fees with her ability.

So even though this is a book for those who do not get insurance through an employer, you still need to understand all the insurance options that are offered. You will find, if you are navigating a public health system (such as Massachusetts' new "everyone must have health insurance" program), that you have to choose between a variety of programs and costs.

As you read about each health-care option and plan, consider what you need as opposed to what you think you can afford. For example:

- ◆ Do you have a doctor you like already, and do you want to find a way to continue seeing him or her?

- ◆ Does your health require consistent care or regular visits to clinics for special attention or testing?

◆ Do you have a preexisting condition that will affect the type of health insurance you can buy?

◆ Are you almost—or already—at the age where you qualify for Medicare?

◆ Do you qualify for Medicaid?

◆ Is your biggest concern not regular health care, such as check-ups, but being covered in case of emergency?

◆ Do you need to worry about care for an entire family?

◆ Would you be comfortable paying cash for some appointments?

As you can see from this list of questions, a number of different situations could determine whether you need health insurance or simply need to figure out a health plan on your own.

Of course, as we will cover in more detail, some people, specifically those in Massachusetts, Maine, and maybe by the time you read this, California, are required to have health insurance, but they still need to decide exactly what type of coverage is best for them.

> **Bet You Didn't Know**
>
> Insurance offered by employers is heavily subsidized by the federal government since it's not taxed as income by individuals.

Getting a Basic Understanding of Health Insurance

For a basic understanding of health insurance it is useful to break insurance policies down into their component parts. These are:

◆ Administration

◆ Network/discount agreements

◆ Actual insurance

In addition to providing a better understanding of the policies, knowing about these components is necessary to better compare and choose among the profusion of different insurance products available.

Administration relates to the rules and regulations of the plan. Who will process the paperwork? Is it a large insurance company (Blue Cross Plan or large national insurer), a "third party administrator," or perhaps your employer? What are the rules and regulations or the plan? Are there co-pays, deductibles, co-insurance? Do you need "pre-approval" for hospitalization or procedures? Do you need referrals from a primary care doctor to see specialists?

Network/discount agreements give you access to a panel of providers who have agreed to a negotiated fee for their services—often a significant discount (in some cases 50 percent or more) off their "list price."

The insurance component is the contracted amount you are actually covered for. This is what the insurer will pay. There will be language which limits the insurer's liability both on an individual occurrence and lifetime basis.

Now that we know the basic components of a health insurance policy we can better evaluate and understand the types of plans available.

Three Basic Insurance Plans

There are three basic types of health insurance plans and endless variations on these types. If you can understand the three types of plans and the three components of each plan, you will have made great progress in your understanding and ability to judge the variety of options.

The three basic types are:

◆ Indemnity insurance plans

◆ Health Maintenance Organization (HMO) plans

◆ Preferred Provider Organization (PPO) plans

Indemnity plans are similar to most commonly available insurance, like life, auto, and homeowner's insurance. The insured has a claim, files with the insurance company, and is reimbursed for the loss. Depending on the provider, the insurance company may pay the doctor or hospital directly, or may pay you, the insured, and then you pay the provider. In the typical straight indemnity plan the provider is free to charge whatever he wants and you are free to negotiate or make whatever agreements you want with the provider.

In an HMO plan you are contracting for both insurance and healthcare with the same entity. The HMO is both the insurer and provider of health care services. Usually you are required to see an HMO doctor who is either a direct employee ("staff model HMO") or contractor ("open model HMO"). In this case you may receive *no* reimbursement for expenses incurred for non-HMO doctors or hospitals.

In a PPO plan there is a "network" of providers with prearranged discount agreements that you now have access to. You can stay within the network and avail yourself of the discounted rates or (usually) go outside the network and pay for care and make whatever agreements you want with "non-network" providers. Reimbursement for out-of-network services is limited by the plan rules and often penalized by a lower plan payment.

The insurance companies mix and match the basic components and plan types together in an endless (and confusing) variety of "products" at a variety of different "price points." You can, for example, buy just a PPO network discount plan at a very cheap rate. You must understand, however, that you are *not* getting insurance and will be personally liable to pay the full fee or you forfeit the discount. There is also inexpensive indemnity insurance available (often through student health plans) which provides for very limited reimbursement that often leaves the "insured" stuck with a *very* large "balance bill," potentially more than the "insurance" payment. At the opposite end of the spectrum there are plans available that provide first-dollar coverage and limitless choice of providers, but come with a *very* large premium payment amount.

My advice is first to try to get some kind of insurance (be it public, employer sponsored, or individual) whenever possible. Any insurance is usually better than no insurance in that it provides you with better access to care. The second piece of advice is to get the best combination of components and plans you can reasonably afford.

Bet You Didn't Know

Even those with employer-based health insurance aren't always covered by the big insurance companies. Many companies, such as Ford and Chrysler, as well as smaller ones, are self-insured. This means they either pay claims themselves or contract for Administrative Services Only (ASO) through a large insurance company, such as Blue Cross. Blue Cross uses the self-insured company's money to pay the claim.

> **Code Red**
>
> The best health insurance plans (and those offered by industrialized countries) are comprehensive (they cover all medically necessary services provided by hospitals and doctors), universal (all insured persons are entitled to uniform terms, conditions, and care), accessible (one's care cannot be impeded by financing or other barriers), and portable (it stays with an individual no matter what her circumstances).

The Value of Choice

Money (or lack of it) is obviously a significant barrier to health care, but opting for the cheaper health plan at the outset can cost in financial ways in the long run. When I was a resident physician, my health insurance options were an HMO based at my hospital and a Point of service (POS/Indemnity) Plan. I chose the latter because I like and value choice, even though it was more expensive upfront. Then, one day while sailing, I tore a cartilage in my knee.

While the HMO had one orthopedic surgeon on staff (who may well have been very good but who I didn't know), a physician I did know recommended an orthopedic surgeon at Northwestern University who happened to be the team physician for the Chicago Bulls. So I went to see him.

When he examined my knee, he said I needed an arthroscopy and then open surgery. When I asked the doctor why he couldn't perform the surgery through the arthroscope he candidly admitted that he hadn't had enough experience with the arthroscope (this was 1979 and it was a very new procedure). So I asked who could and the doctor gave me the names of five doctors in the entire United States who could do the procedure (at that time).

When I called the nearest expert, his secretary asked if I was calling to sign up for his arthroscopy course. I knew I had found the right doctor. I flew to Detroit and had the surgery with a much shorter recovery than the old open/non-arthroscopic procedure. In fact, it was the difference of several weeks recovery versus close to a year.

Now, this example is relatively trivial, but had this been a life or death situation, choice might have been much more important. There was no difference in price and, in fact, when I did this, I was a "poor resident" with income of about $15,000 annually. I paid the $79 airfare myself and flew home immediately on discharge to avoid a hotel bill. It was well worth it.

In this example, choice was a factor in quality of care, but there was no difference in price.

While all the doctors in these various plans theoretically have their patients' best interests at heart, it is important to understand the financial incentives and thus the potential for subliminal (or not so subliminal) bias. In the Indemnity/PPO/POS models, the doctor's financial incentive is to do (and bill for) as much as possible. In the HMO model, the incentive is to keep people healthy and provide cost-effective care. There is, however, also an incentive to avoid hospitalizations, specialty referrals, and more expensive tests and treatments.

So, now that you have a better understanding of your options, read the contract carefully, and choose your poison.

Public and Private Healthcare

According to Physicians for A National Health Program, an organization of doctors advocating for a single-payer health program, the United States spends more on health care than any other industrialized nation, about $7,129 per person each year. Unfortunately, most of this money is spent in administrative costs. The cost of health insurance paperwork consumes 31 percent of every health-care dollar.

By my own estimate (a wild guess based on my observation of my own practice and that of my colleagues) as much as 25 percent (or more) of every healthcare dollar goes for "defensive medicine" to prevent malpractice lawsuits. The Institute of Medicine (IOM) disagrees with me and puts this latter figure at about 3 percent. I think (of course) that my figure is closer to the truth. If I am right then well more than 51 percent of every healthcare dollar goes to pay for something besides necessary healthcare.

Currently, the United States is a mix of public and private health insurance and health care. Some of us use the public health system, funded through the federal and state government, to find doctors and pay for care, while others of us use private insurance companies, such as Kaiser Permanente, Blue Cross/Blue Shield, and Humana to help pay for our care.

Government insurance, such as Medicare and Medicaid, is available to certain individuals under specific circumstances. Medicare is the health-care plan for US citizens aged 65 years or older, persons with disabilities, and those with chronic renal failure. However, most individuals need secondary insurance coverage to help with expenses not covered by Medicare. Recently, Medicare has developed prescription drug coverage to assist senior citizens with the cost of prescribed medications. Medicaid is health insurance for persons with very low incomes and for the disabled who do not qualify for Medicare. Each state has strict criteria for Medicaid qualification.

Also most states have their own medical assistance plan that allows lower-income citizens, who would otherwise be unable to afford health care, get covered. These plans aren't always free.

Healthcare Options for Active Duty and Retired Military Personnel

Most Americans believe that anyone who has served our country in the military gets free medical care for life, but in 2007, a government panel found that almost two million veterans were uninsured. And those who were insured often had inferior mental health coverage, even when they were coming home from Iraq or other combat situations. Veterans 65 and older are eligible for Medicare.

In fact, about 12.7 percent of nonelderly veterans—or one in eight—lacked health coverage in 2004, the most recent year for which figures are available.

TRICARE

TRICARE is the Department of Defense's worldwide health-care program for active duty and retired uniformed services members and their families. It consists of TRICARE Prime, a *managed care* option; TRICARE Extra, a preferred provider option; and TRICARE

Standard, a fee-for-service option. TRICARE For Life is also available for Medicare-eligible beneficiaries age 65 and over.

def•i•ni•tion

Most people think **managed care** and health maintenance organizations (HMOs) are the same thing, but that's not true. Managed care refers to a program in which the insurer has rules that specify which services are covered and which are not. This may defacto dictate which services the doctor or hospital is willing to provide.

According to the TRICARE website, "active duty service members are required to enroll in Prime. Active duty family members, retirees and their family members are encouraged, but not required, to enroll in Prime. However, to receive the TRICARE Prime benefit, they must reside where TRICARE Prime is offered ... TRICARE Prime offers less out-of-pocket costs than any other TRICARE option."

Active duty members and their families do not pay enrollment fees, annual deductibles, or co-payments for care in the TRICARE network. Retired service members pay an annual enrollment fee of $230 for an individual or $460 for a family, and minimal co-pays apply for care in the TRICARE network. TRICARE Prime offers a "point-of-service" option for care received outside of the TRICARE Prime network, but point-of-service care requires payment of significant out-of-pocket costs.

TRICARE Extra is a preferred provider option (PPO) in which beneficiaries choose a doctor, hospital, or other medical provider within the TRICARE provider network.

TRICARE Standard is a fee-for-service option. You can see an authorized TRICARE provider of your choice, but having this flexibility means that care generally costs more.

When beneficiaries age 65 and over become eligible for Medicare Part A, they can use TRICARE For Life (TFL) if they purchase Medicare Part B.

The Veterans Administration

The Veteran's Administration provides health benefits and services to any veteran of the Armed Services. To be eligible:

◆ You must have been in active military service in the army, navy, air force, marines, or coast guard (or merchant marines during WW II).

◆ You must not have received a dishonorable discharge.

Likewise, reservists and National Guard members who serve in a theater of combat operations have special eligibility for medical services, inpatient care, and nursing home care for two years following their discharge.

The Veteran's Administration also offers limited benefits to some family members of service veterans, including The Civilian Health And Medical Program of Veterans Affairs (CHAMPVA). CHAMPVA offers help to spouses and children of veterans who have been determined as permanently and totally disabled due to a service-connected disability, the surviving spouse or children of veterans who died from a VA-rated service connected disability, the surviving spouse or children of a veteran who (at the time of death) was considered permanently and totally disabled from a service connected disability, or the surviving spouse or child of military personnel who died in the line of duty. Call 1-800-733-8387.

> **Bet You Didn't Know**
>
> The VA has a spina bifida program that covers costs for children of Vietnam or Korean veterans who served from September 1, 1967 and August 31, 1971 and who were exposed to herbicide in the DMZ. This is not a full health-care program, and those who qualify must have a diagnosis of spina bifida.

Nearly eight million veterans were enrolled in the VA health system in 2006, but that number doesn't include "Priority 8 veterans," who have no service-connected disabilities and whose earnings generally are above 80 percent of the median income where they live. Congress held hearings in 2007 to see if Priority 8 veterans should be added to the health-care rolls because so many of these veterans do not have health care.

If the Veteran's Administration were to add these soldiers to the budget, experts believe it would cost from $366 million to $3.3 billion annually. However, especially since we are at war as of this writing, many representatives believe all veterans should be cared for. "All veterans should have access to 'their' health-care system. [Not giving these veterans coverage] is rationing health care to veterans, those who have served our nation. And I think it's unacceptable for a nation of our wealth and our ability," said Rep. Bob Filner (D-Calif.).

But, on the other hand, Rep. Steve Buyer (Ind.), said Veterans Affairs should focus on its "core constituency"—veterans with service-related health problems, the indigent, and those with "catastrophic" disabilities. "Some say the government is obliged to provide essentially free health care for life to anyone who served even a year or two," he said. "I intend to protect the core constituency first."

Keep in mind that these two gentlemen, as Congressmen, are entitled to a lifetime of free health care as are their families—even if they serve only one term.

State by State Health Insurance Options

According to a report published by The Urban Institute (January 2002), "access (to health care) for the uninsured can vary considerably across states and communities." The *safety net*, which is designed to help those who are uninsured, is greatly affected by "states' uninsured rates, marketplace competition, Medicaid payment policies, and state and local financial support," because all of these considerations "exert pressure on the safety net."

def•i•ni•tion

The **safety net** is an amalgam of programs, services, and organizations designed to ensure that no American goes without care. Unfortunately, the safety net is not a guarantee of good care. More problematic, however, is the idea that Americans shouldn't need a safety net and thus working Americans are often priced out of both social services and health insurance—leaving them without a safety net at all.

While much of the structure of the safety net is laid out by the federal government in the form of Medicaid, the true day-to-day appearance of the program varies from state to state. In some locations, the services are entirely run by government departments; in others, it's a mix of private and public funds.

The insurance industry stresses the safety net system as much as it stresses individuals. Because, ironically, states who have fewer insured citizens, such as California, Texas, and Florida, are more likely to have more patients who can't pay anything toward their health care than those states who have more insured patients. In other words, no insurance often means no money at all for medical care. In fact, according to a report published by The Access Project in 2003, these safety net resources, such as public hospitals, are rarely free. One in five, in fact, did not offer reduced rates to uninsured people.

According to a report by Norton & Lipson (1998), California, Texas, and Florida have the most vulnerable safety nets; Alabama, Mississippi, New York, and New Jersey are somewhat vulnerable; while Minnesota, Washington, and Wisconsin are the least vulnerable.

Massachusetts was on the least vulnerable list, but since then, they became the first state to institute mandatory health-care insurance for all residents. Meanwhile, most likely because of its status as a most vulnerable state, California's governor, Arnold Schwarzenegger, proposed extending health-care coverage to all of California's 36 million residents.

California

One-fifth of California's population, or 6.5 million people, do not have health insurance, which is an amount far higher than in any other state. Less than half of California workers get health insurance through their jobs, according to a study set for release today. The rest find coverage through a partner or spouse, a government program, or are uninsured.

The study by the Center on Policy Initiatives, a San Diego nonprofit that researches issues affecting workers, found that 49 percent of working Californians receive coverage through their employers, while 15 percent have insurance through somebody else, typically a spouse or partner.

At least one million of the uninsured are illegal immigrants, state officials say.

The plan, which Mr. Schwarzenegger estimated would cost $12 billion, calls for many employers who do not offer health insurance to contribute to a fund that would help pay for coverage of the working uninsured. It would also require doctors to pay 2 percent and hospitals 4 percent of their revenues to help cover higher reimbursements for those who treat patients enrolled in Medi-Cal, the state's Medicaid program.

Under Mr. Schwarzenegger's proposal, Medi-Cal would be extended to adults who earn as much as 100 percent above the federal poverty line and to children, regardless of their immigration status, living in homes where the family income is as much as 300 percent above that line, about $60,000 a year for a family of four.

Most states follow federal health insurance guidelines to a large extent—for example, HIPAA laws (see Chapter 1), COBRA laws, and other nondiscrimination regulations.

Local Coverage

Because health insurance is such an overwhelming issue that federal or state governments have not adequately handled, some municipalities, especially those overwhelmed by uninsured citizens, such as San Francisco, are taking the matter into their own hands.

In June 2006, Gavin Newsom, San Francisco's mayor, announced a plan that would provide comprehensive health care for all San Francisco residents. Called The San Francisco Health Care Security Ordinance, the plan provides health care (not health insurance) for anyone who falls well below the poverty level and who has no other health insurance. It will cover prescriptions, doctor visits, and mental health care but not dental or vision care.

The program will cost about $200 million; some individuals will have to pay premiums, but local employers will contribute the most to the plan. As you can imagine, many small business employers are fighting this. Restaurants, for example, often only have a profit margin of 3 percent, which makes covering health insurance premiums for staffers virtually a guaranteed way to shut down a business.

The States

Each state has numerous different laws and regulations that cover health insurance, including specific details on one's rights as an employee, as a low-income resident, or as a person with disabilities. Likewise, all state residents are also offered protections from the federal government, using a variety of programs, including HIPAA, the Family and Medical Leave Act, and others. Not every eligible health-care and health-insurance right is covered in this list as it is only meant to be an introduction.

To get the information and help you need takes a fair amount of research and phone calls and paperwork, but it is possible. And it is also true that most states report that many of their residents do not take advantage of the assistance offered to them, often because they don't know about it. So pick up the phone and start asking questions.

For Your Health

To read complete information about each state's coverage and the rights of its citizens, go to www.healthinsuranceinfo. net/guides_map.htm. The information below is provided by the Health Policy Institute of Georgetown University.

When you call, remember to ask the name of the person with whom you are speaking, noting, too, the date and time you speak with her. Take notes on what she tells you, and request to speak to the same person each time you call.

Alabama

Private insurers commonly offer fee-for-service payment plans in Alabama, while the state offers The Alabama Health Insurance Plan. You can join this program, run by Blue Cross Blue Shield, if you are HIPAA eligible but have no other insurance coverage, including COBRA or private insurance. Your premiums will be based on your coverage level, your age and sex, as well as whether or not you smoke. In January, the monthly premiums for a 24-year-old nonsmoking male ranged from $149 to $195 while the monthly premiums for a 64-year-old, nonsmoking man were $495 to $646. Premiums increase each year with age. Call 1-800-513-1834 or 334-352-8924.

Alaska

If you do not have coverage through an employer, you may be able to buy an individual health insurance policy from the Alaska Comprehensive Health Insurance Association (ACHIA). You will not have a preexisting condition exclusion period, and there are limits on what you can be charged for an ACHIA policy. You may also be able to buy insurance from ACHIA if you have had difficulty obtaining affordable health insurance from private companies because of your health condition. In this case you may face a new preexisting condition exclusion period. The Alaska Medicaid program offers free health coverage for pregnant women, families with children, the elderly, and disabled individuals with very low incomes. Call 907-465-5824.

Bet You Didn't Know

Web searches, using Google, Yahoo, and other search engines, are a great way to get some basic information on your rights as a state citizen. Type in the name of your state; then use words such as health care, individual coverage, or health programs. Bookmark all sites that give information you need, and use this info when you call the state for coverage or assistance.

Arizona

If you are an employer with 50 or fewer employees, including the self-employed, you may be eligible to obtain coverage through the Healthcare Group of Arizona (HCGA) if you meet certain requirements. For HCGA, call 602-417-6755 or 800-247-2289.

Arkansas

Generally, in Arkansas, no limits exist on how much individual premiums can vary due to age, gender, health status, family size, and other factors. Some citizens can buy individual health insurance from the Arkansas Comprehensive Health Insurance Pool (CHIP), the Arkansas subsidized health coverage for pregnant women, families with children, elderly, and disabled individuals with very low incomes. CHIP coverage is offered through a managed care plan. After you satisfy your annual deductible, the plan will pay 80 percent of covered charges when you get care from a hospital, doctor, or other provider in the CHIP network. For (CHIP) Program/Arkansas Blue Cross Blue Shield (plan administrator), call 1-800-998-7542.

California

If you have had difficulty obtaining affordable individual health insurance because of your health condition, you may be eligible for Major Risk Medical Insurance Program (MRMIP). When you exhaust MRMIP coverage (36 months), you will be guaranteed a health insurance policy in the individual market. You will not face a new preexisting condition exclusion period, and there are limits on what you can be charged for this policy. If you have low or modest household income, you may be eligible for free or subsidized health coverage for yourself or members of your family through Medi-Cal, which offers free health coverage for pregnant women, families with children, elderly and disabled individuals with very low incomes. If your children are 18 years old or younger, do not have health insurance, and meet other qualifications, they may be eligible to buy health insurance through the Healthy Families Program. For MRMIP, call 916-324-4695; for California Department of Health Services, 916-636-1980.

Connecticut

If you lose your group health plan and meet other qualifications, you can buy individual health insurance from the Connecticut Health Reinsurance Association (HRA). You will not face a new preexisting condition exclusion period. If you have low or modest household income but are not eligible for Medicaid, your children may be eligible for free or low-cost health insurance through the Healthcare for Uninsured Kids (HUSKY) program. For HRA, call 1-800-842-0004 and for the State of Connecticut Department of Social Services (for HUSKY), call 1-877-284-8759.

Colorado

If you lose your group health plan and meet other qualifications, you can buy an individual health insurance policy from CoverColorado.

You will not have a preexisting condition exclusion period. For CoverColorado, call 1-888-461-3811.

Delaware

Other than Medicaid and the Delaware Healthy Children Program, little is available for insurance or health care in Delaware. Call Delaware Health and Social Services at 1-800-464-4357.

Florida

Other than Medicaid, Florida offers little assistance to those without insurance. One program is Florida KidCare, which provides health coverage to low-income families with children under the age of 19 who are not eligible for Medicaid and who are uninsured or underinsured. Call 1-888-540-5437.

Georgia

The Georgia Medicaid program offers free health coverage for pregnant women, families with children, elderly and disabled individuals with very low incomes while Georgia PeachCare for Kids provides health coverage to low-income Georgia children under the age of 19 who are not eligible for Medicaid and who have limited or no health insurance. Call the Georgia Department of Community Health at 1-877-GA-PEACH.

Hawaii

The Hawaii Medicaid program includes the Medicaid Fee-for-Service Program and Hawaii QUEST, which offers free health coverage for pregnant women, families with children, and elderly and disabled individuals with very low incomes. Hawaii Quest also offers free or subsidized health insurance for some low-income Hawaii residents who are not eligible for Medicaid. Call Hawaii Department of Human Services at 808-586-5390.

Idaho

Idaho residents are guaranteed the right to buy Individual High Risk Reinsurance Pool (HRP) plans under certain circumstances. You may be able to buy an HRP plan if an Idaho insurer turns you down due to health status or claims experience or offers to sell you coverage at a premium higher than that charged for HRP plans. You cannot be charged more for an HRP plan coverage due to your health status. Call the Idaho Department of Insurance at 208-334-4250.

Illinois

If you lose your group health plan and meet other qualifications, you can buy an individual health insurance policy from the Illinois Comprehensive Health Insurance Plan (CHIP). If your children are 18 years old or younger and meet certain financial qualifications, you may be able to buy insurance for them or receive assistance paying for private health insurance through the Illinois All Kids/KidCare Program. For CHIP, call the State Health Benefits Risk Pool at 1-800-962-8384; for Illinois All Kids/Kidcare, call the Illinois Department of Public Aid at 1-866-255-5437.

Indiana

If you lose your group health plan and meet other qualifications, you can buy an individual health insurance policy from the Indiana Comprehensive Health Insurance Association (ICHIA). You will not have a preexisting condition exclusion period. You may also be able to buy insurance from ICHIA if you have had difficulty obtaining affordable health insurance from private companies because of your health condition. In this case you may face a new preexisting condition exclusion period. There are limits on what you can be charged for an ICHIA policy. Call ICHIA at 1-800-552-7921.

Iowa

If you are HIPAA eligible or have been denied individual insurance because of your health status, you can buy coverage from the Iowa

Comprehensive Health Association (HIP-IOWA). There are limits on what you can be charged for an HIP-IOWA policy; however, depending on how you become eligible, you may face a new preexisting condition exclusion period. If your child is 19 years or younger, does not have health insurance, and meets other qualifications, you may be able to receive low cost or free health insurance for them through the Healthy and Well Kids in Iowa (hawk-I) program. For HIP-IOWA coverage, call 1-877-793-6880; for hawk-I, call 1-800-257-8563.

Kansas

If you lose your group health insurance and meet other qualifications, you can buy an individual health plan from the Kansas Health Insurance Association (KHIA). The Kansas Medicaid program offers free health coverage for pregnant women, families with children, elderly and disabled individuals with very low incomes. If your children are under age 19, do not have health insurance, and meet other qualifications, you may be able to buy insurance for them through HealthWave. Call Kansas Health Insurance Association (KHIA) Benefit Management, Inc. at 1-800-290-1368; for HealthWave, call the Division of Health Care Policy, Kansas Department of Social and Rehabilitation Services, at 1-800-792-4884.

Kentucky

If you lose your group health insurance coverage, you can buy individual health insurance from Kentucky Access. For Kentucky Access, call 1-866-405-6145.

Louisiana

If you lose your group health insurance and meet other qualifications, you may be able to buy individual health insurance coverage from the Louisiana Health Plan (LHP). You can also buy insurance from LHP if you have been a Louisiana resident for six months and have been turned down by two health insurance companies or you are not able to obtain coverage below a certain premium and meet other qualifications.). Call LHP at 225-926-6245.

Maine

Maine was the first state (in 2003) to approve universal health coverage for all citizens, but, surprisingly, it has had fewer enrollees than expected. The DirigoChoice plan offers insurance to people on a sliding scale. But young, healthy people have not enrolled the way they need to in order to make the program successful. Instead, large numbers of those who need subsidies have enrolled. Maine does not allow insurance companies to offer discounts on premiums to large companies or to deny coverage to anyone, which has meant that the price of premiums are very high and the number of insurance providers has decreased. Most citizens view this as a form of over-regulation that has made their ability to get insurance more problematic. Call 207-287-9900.

Maryland

If you lose your group health insurance and meet other qualifications, you can buy an individual health insurance policy from the Maryland Health Insurance Plan (MHIP). You will not face a new preexisting condition exclusion period if you are HIPAA eligible, and there are limits on what you can be charged for a high risk pool policy. If you have had difficulty obtaining an affordable individual health insurance policy because of your health condition, you may also be eligible under MHIP. You will not face a new preexisting condition exclusion period. There are limits on what you can be charged for a high risk pool policy, too. For MHIP, call 1-866-780-7150; for MCHP Premium, call the Maryland Department of Health and Mental Hygiene at 1-800-456-8900.

Massachusetts

Massachusetts now requires all residents to carry health insurance. To find out which program would be best for you, go to www.mahealthconnector.org.

Michigan

All Michigan residents are guaranteed the right to buy an individual health policy from Blue Cross Blue Shield of Michigan. You will not face a new preexisting condition exclusion period, nor will you be charged more due to your health status, age, or any other factor. In addition, HMOs in Michigan are also required to offer all products to all individuals on a guaranteed issue basis during one annual 30-day open enrollment period. If you are self-employed, you can qualify to buy small group health insurance from Blue Cross Blue Shield of Michigan. Blue Cross Blue Shield must sell "group of one" policies to sole proprietors. Call Blue Cross Blue Shield of Michigan at 313-225-8100.

Bet You Didn't Know

Have you noticed how each state has its own coverage regulations and programs to help its citizens? Americans do not have portable insurance like those in other industrialized countries do. When an American moves or changes jobs, her insurance changes with her. And some Americans move to certain states, such as senior citizens to Florida, because of the way the state protects health insurance rights. However, when one group is protected, another is often neglected. Children in Florida, for example, do not get the benefits that the elderly do.

Minnesota

If you lose your group health plan and meet other qualifications, you can buy coverage from the Minnesota Comprehensive Health Association (MCHA high-risk pool. You will not face a new preexisting condition exclusion period. There are limits on what you can be charged for MCHA coverage. You can also buy coverage from MCHA if you have a serious health condition or if you have been turned down by a health insurance company. In this case you may face a new preexisting condition exclusion period. MCHA 1-866-894-8053.

Mississippi

If you lose your group health insurance and meet other qualifications, you can buy an individual health plan from the Mississippi Comprehensive Health Insurance Risk Pool Association (MCHIRPA). You will not face a new preexisting condition exclusion period. There are limits on what you can be charged for an MCHIRPA policy. If you have had difficulty obtaining affordable individual health insurance because of your health condition, you may also be eligible for MCHIRPA coverage. In this case you may face a new preexisting condition exclusion period, but there are limits on what you can be charged for an MCHIRPA policy. For MCHIRPA-Blue Cross/Blue Shield of Mississippi (plan administrator), call 601-362-0799.

Missouri

You can buy insurance from the Missouri Health Insurance Pool (MHIP) if you have had difficulty obtaining affordable health insurance from private companies because of your health condition. In this case you may face a new preexisting condition exclusion period. There are limits on what you can be charged for an MHIP policy. Call MHIP at 1-800-821-2231.

Montana

If you lose your group health plan and meet other qualifications, you can buy individual health insurance from the Montana Comprehensive Health Association (MCHA) high-risk pool. All your preexisting conditions will be covered immediately under the benefits provided. Premiums will vary based on your age. You can also buy insurance from MCHA if you have been turned down by at least two health insurance companies or have a serious health condition and meet other qualifications. In this case you may face a new preexisting condition exclusion period if you haven't had coverage lately. Call MCHA at 1-800-447-7828.

Nebraska

If you lose your group health insurance and meet other qualifications, you can buy individual health insurance from the Nebraska Comprehensive Health Insurance Pool (CHIP). You will not face a new preexisting condition exclusion period. You can also buy insurance from CHIP if you have been turned down by a health insurance company and meet other qualifications. Call CHIP at 402-390-1814.

Bet You Didn't Know

While every state has different regulations (that change often), here are some reasons you might be considered "uninsurable" and thus eligible for a public insurance program: you are HIV positive; you have disability and are eligible for Medicare; you have been turned down for coverage by two or more insurance companies; your insurance premium has increased by more than 50 percent, or, because of another risk factor, your premium is 50 percent more than that of someone who is a standard risk.

Nevada

If your children are 18 years old or younger, do not have health insurance, and meet other qualifications, you may be able to buy insurance for them through the Nevada Check Up program. Call 1-877-543-7669.

New Hampshire

If you lose your group health plan and meet other qualifications, you can buy health insurance from the New Hampshire Health Plan (NHHP). You will not face a new preexisting condition exclusion period if you are HIPAA eligible. There are limits on what you can be charged for this health insurance. If you are not HIPAA eligible and have had difficulty obtaining affordable individual health insurance because of your health condition, you may also be eligible for health insurance from the NHHP. Call NHHP 1-877-888-6447.

New Jersey

In New Jersey, if your children are 18 years old and younger, are uninsured, and meet certain eligibility requirements, they may be eligible for health insurance through NJ Family Care. Call 1-800-701-0710.

New Mexico

If you lose your group health plan and meet other qualifications, you can buy individual health insurance from the New Mexico Medical Insurance Pool (NMMIP) or from the New Mexico Health Insurance

Alliance (the Alliance). You will not have a preexisting condition exclusion period. There are limits on what you can be charged for coverage under NMMIP and the Alliance.

If you are not HIPAA eligible but have difficulty obtaining an affordable individual health insurance policy because of your health condition, you may also be eligible for NMMIP coverage. Call New Mexico Health Insurance Alliance at 505-989-1600; for NMMIP, call Blue Cross and Blue Shield of New Mexico at 505-816-4248.

New York

The Child Health Plus Program offers free or subsidized health coverage for uninsured children. In addition, the Family Health Plus Program offers free health coverage for eligible uninsured families and individuals. The Healthy New York program offers low-cost health insurance to uninsured working individuals, small employers, and sole-proprietors. For Child Health Plus New York, call the Department of Health at 1-800-698-4543; for Family Health Plus, call 1-877-9FHPLUS (1-877-934-7587); for Healthy New York, call 1-866-HEALTHY NY (1-866-432-5849).

North Carolina

North Carolina Health Choice for Children is a state-designed program that provides health coverage to low-income children under the age of 19 who are not eligible for Medicaid and who have limited or no health insurance. Call 1-800-367-2229.

North Dakota

If you lose your group health insurance and meet other qualifications, you can buy individual health insurance from the Comprehensive Health Association of North Dakota (CHAND) high-risk pool or under a group conversion policy. You will not face a new preexisting condition exclusion period. There are limits on what you can be charged for a CHAND policy. You can also buy insurance from CHAND if you have been turned down or excluded for certain coverage by a health insurance company and meet other qualifications. In this case you may face a new preexisting condition exclusion period. For CHAND Blue Cross Blue Shield of North Dakota, call 1-800-737-0016; for Healthy Steps, 701-328-2321.

Ohio

Ohio's Best Rx Program is a prescription drug discount card program designed to lower the cost of prescription for eligible residents. Call 614-466-9783.

Oklahoma

If you lose your group health insurance and meet other qualifications, you can buy an individual health insurance policy from the Oklahoma Health Insurance High-Risk Pool. You will not face a new preexisting condition exclusion period. There are limits on what you can be charged for a High-Risk Pool policy. If you have had difficulty obtaining affordable individual health insurance because of your health condition, you may also be eligible for High-Risk Pool coverage. In this case you may face a new preexisting condition exclusion period. SoonerCare offers free or subsidized health coverage for pregnant women, families with children, elderly and disabled individuals with very low incomes. Call Oklahoma Health Insurance High Risk Pool Epoch Group (plan administrator) at 1-800-255-6065, x4767; for SoonerCare, call 1-800-987-7767.

Oregon

If you have been denied individual coverage because of your health status, you can buy individual coverage from the Oregon Medical Insurance Pool (OMIP). In this case you will pay a premium surcharge and may have a preexisting condition exclusion period.

If you have low or modest household income, you may be eligible for the Family Health Insurance Assistance Program (FHIAP), which subsidizes health insurance premiums for qualified Oregonians. For OMIP Oregon Blue Cross Blue Shield (plan administrator), call 503-373-1692 for FHIAP, 503-373-1692.

Pennsylvania

If you lose your group health plan and meet other qualifications, you can buy an individual health policy from a Blue Cross Blue Shield plan operating in your region of Pennsylvania. You will not face a new pre-existing condition exclusion period. Blue Cross and Blue Shield must offer you a choice of at least two policies, including one with comprehensive benefits. If you are not HIPAA eligible, Blue Cross and Blue Shield plans operating in Pennsylvania must offer you at least one individual health insurance policy on a guaranteed issue basis. You cannot be turned down for this policy because you are sick.

If you have low or modest household income, you may be eligible for subsidized health coverage through a state-run program called AdultBasic. For Highmark Blue Cross Blue Shield, call 1-800-544-6679; Blue Cross of Northeastern Pennsylvania and Blue Shield, 1-800-829-8599; AdultBasic Health Insurance Program, 800-GO-BASIC.

Rhode Island

No state programs are available in Rhode Island, aside from Medicaid. Call 401-462-5300.

South Carolina

If you lose your group health insurance and meet other qualifications, you can buy individual health coverage from the South Carolina Health Insurance Pool (SCHIP). You will not face a new preexisting condition exclusion period. There are limits on what you can be charged for a SCHIP policy. If you have had difficulty obtaining affordable individual health insurance because of your health condition, you may also be eligible for SCHIP coverage. In this case you may face a new preexisting condition exclusion period. There are limits on what you can be charged for a SCHIP policy. For SCHIP Blue Cross and Blue Shield (SCHIP administrator), call 1-800-868-2500; for Medicaid, call 1-888-549-0820.

South Dakota

If you have had at least 12 months of creditable coverage and then lose it, you may be guaranteed the right to buy a policy from the South

Dakota Risk Pool. You will not face a new pre-existing condition exclusion period. There are limits on what you can be charged for a high risk pool policy. Call the South Dakota Risk Pool at 605-773-3148.

Tennessee

If you apply to buy individual health insurance from a private insurer and are turned down or if you have a qualifying health condition, you can buy health insurance from the Tennessee high-risk pool, AccessTN. CoverTN is a state-sponsored program that provides small employers access to health insurance at a reduced premium. If you have low or modest household income, you may be eligible for free or subsidized health coverage for yourself or members of your family. TennCare offers free or subsidized health coverage for pregnant women, families with children, elderly and disabled individuals with very low incomes. For TennCare, 1-866-311-4287.

Texas

If you lose your group health plan and meet other qualifications, you can buy an individual health insurance policy from the Texas Health Insurance Risk Pool. You will not face a new preexisting condition exclusion period. There are limits on what you can be charged for a Health Pool policy. The Texas Children's Health Insurance Program (CHIP) offers subsidized health coverage for certain uninsured children. For Texas Health Insurance Risk Pool (Health Pool) Blue Cross/Blue Shield of Texas (plan administrator), call 1-888-398-3927; for CHIP, 1-800-647-6558.

Utah

If you lose your group health plan and meet other qualifications, you can buy individual health insurance either from the Utah Comprehensive Health Insurance Pool (HIPUtah) or an individual market insurer. There are limits on what you can be charged for a HIPUtah policy. If you apply to buy individual health insurance from a private insurer and are turned down, you can buy health insurance from HIPUtah. Because HIPUtah covers only very sick individuals, if you do not qualify as a high health risk, you will be given a certificate of insurability that will guarantee you the right to buy an individual health insurance policy from a private insurance company. Call HIPUtah SelectHealth (plan administrator) at 801-442-5038; for CHIP, 1-888-222-2542.

Vermont

If your children are 18 years old or younger, do not have health insurance, and meet other qualifications, you may be able to buy insurance for them through a program called Dr. Dynasaur. Call 1-800-250-8427.

Virginia

All residents are guaranteed the right to buy individual health insurance from either Anthem Blue Cross Blue Shield or CareFirst Blue Cross Blue Shield, depending on where you live. For Anthem Blue Cross Blue Shield, call 1-800-552-7945.

Washington

The Washington State Health Insurance Pool (WSHIP) is available to residents. Call 1-800-877-5187.

West Virginia

You have the right to buy individual health insurance from AccessWV. You will not face a new preexisting condition exclusion period. There are limits on what you can be charged for an AccessWV policy. Call the West Virginia Insurance Commission at 1-800-624-9004.

Wisconsin

You can buy individual health insurance from the Health Insurance Risk Sharing Plan (HIRSP). HIRSP provides insurance coverage for residents of Wisconsin who, because of health conditions, are unable to obtain private health insurance and for people who are HIPAA eligible. Call HIRSP 1-800-828-4777.

Wyoming

You can buy an individual health insurance policy from the Wyoming Health Insurance Pool (WHIP). Call the Wyoming Department of Health at 307-777-7656; Blue Cross and Blue Shield of Wyoming (WHIP administrator) at 307-634-1393.

Getting Healthcare When You Are Already Sick Versus When You Are Healthy

Unfortunately, all the information described above is more theoretical than practical if you have no insurance and are sick right now. As we mentioned in Chapter 1, many insurance plans have existing conditions riders, which means that if you try to buy insurance having had—or being still challenged by—a serious illness or injury, you may not be able to buy the insurance you want.

Figuring Out Which Plan You Need

Sometimes it is difficult for consumers to purchase insurance or make good health-care choices because they have a rough idea of how much they can spend, but they don't put the actual numbers down on paper. Likewise, they may not stop to really understand their medical needs.

Use this worksheet to determine exactly what you want to buy in terms of coverage. To get started, get out your medical bills from last year or a year in which you had the coverage that helped the most. Don't just include what you spent out-of-pocket. If you had employer-based coverage into which you contributed from your paycheck, include that monthly or bi-monthly deduction.

This form will allow you to compare three policies and give you an idea of what to look for when asking insurance salesmen about their products.

	Policy #1	Policy #2	Policy #3
Monthly Premium (multiply by four for annual cost)	_____	_____	_____
Individual? Family?	_____	_____	_____
Deductible?	_____	_____	_____
Co-payment rate?	_____	_____	_____
Mental Health Rate?	_____	_____	_____
Dental Rate?	_____	_____	_____
Annual Limits on care?	_____	_____	_____
Is there a maximum out-of-pocket cost?	_____	_____	_____
Total yearly estimated cost?	_____	_____	_____

The Least You Need to Know

◆ Finding a doctor whom you like and with whom you are comfortable is more important than picking an insurance plan first.

◆ Many kinds of insurance plans are available, so it's important to choose the one that will give you the most coverage for the most reasonable cost.

◆ Being a veteran does not guarantee that you will receive a lifetime of health care.

◆ Every state has its own regulations regarding insurance and insurance rights as well as coverage for those who can't afford private insurance. You should look into what your state will do for individuals who need help with health care and its associated costs.

Chapter 3

The Information You Need to Get What You Need

In This Chapter

- ◆ Financial, medical, and insurance records
- ◆ The problem with part-time work and insurance coverage
- ◆ The rights of nonmarried partners (of all orientations), widows, and children
- ◆ Ways to be a health-care advocate

As mentioned in Chapter 1, the main reason the United States health insurance system is the most expensive in the world is not because of better medical care but the mounds of paperwork involved and "defensive medicine" to protect against malpractice litigation. As anyone who has ever been to the doctor knows, nothing is more monotonous, annoying, and time-wasting than having to write your name, address, social security number, and allergies each time you go to see a new physician.

Nevertheless, at this point in our system, you have to do this in order to get the care you need. But, wait, it gets worse—or at least more complicated— if you don't have insurance and you're trying to get health care and have a third party, such as a government-subsidized program, pay for your care because a lot more paperwork and record-keeping is required. You won't just need medical records but financial records as well.

The paperwork will become even more cumbersome if you want to care for or help take care of another person, such as your child, a parent, or a sick friend. Plus the mounds of paperwork will exponentially compound if you want to cover a domestic partner or if, unfortunately, you lose a spouse through whom you have been getting your health coverage.

Previous Insurance Records

Most state-run insurance plans that are non-Medicaid related require you to prove you once had group health insurance (typically through an employer) but that you are no longer eligible for it (because of job loss, for example). You will have to show that you cannot afford or are no longer eligible for COBRA.

> **Code Red**
>
> Lying on medical insurance forms is not a good idea. It may come back to haunt you later on as the insurer can legally use this as an excuse for termination of coverage and nonpayment of claims—even for problems unrelated to the issues of untruth on your application.

Private insurers will not ask about your previous insurers, but government insurance, such as programs offered through Unemployment or in a high-risk pool, will. But private insurers will ask for extensive health records, especially in regard to previously diagnosed or chronic medical conditions.

To get private insurance, government-subsidized insurance or health care, financial assistance from providers, or entry into other health-care and insurance programs for you or someone else, you will need (at minimum):

- ◆ Social security numbers for yourself and anyone else on the application
- ◆ The name and address of your previous insurers

- ◆ Your policy numbers

- ◆ A list of any claims you made

- ◆ The reason you stopped using this health insurance policy

- ◆ Verification from the insurance company that your coverage began and started on certain dates

- ◆ Your medical records

What Your Medical Record Should Look Like

You need your medical records both for better health care (to give to your doctor) and for insurance coverage (in case the insurance company wants to know your health history).

Compile these yourself—or better yet, have a knowledgeable health professional (doctor or nurse) do it for you. Start by listing your child-hood vaccination records. Next, list active health conditions, then past history, including surgeries and all diagnoses from the past. Do not keep secrets from your doctor because it could be hazardous to your health.

List all current medications and any allergies to medications (make sure it is a true allergy according to your doctor and not just a drug side effect or intolerance).

Now go the next step. Put this record in a medical style format (to make it easy for the doctor to find what he or she needs) on your com-puter (see the following example medical record). Update it periodically, and mark the date. Save it on your computer, and print a paper copy to bring with you to the doctor. You can even store it on your e-mail server (to make it available anywhere) or carry it in your pocket in a computer memory card or stick. If you don't have a computer, typed or even hand-written records are better than none at all.

If you're really savvy, you will include imaged copies of your most recent EKG, chest X-ray, or other pertinent studies, especially if they are not completely normal.

MEDICAL RECORD SUMMARY
updated as of 7/17/08

NAME: John J. Doe

DOB: 1/17/1954

MEDICAL INSURANCE: AAA Best Health, Policy #50012345;
1-800-454-5105

DOCTORS

William Goodoctor, MD (Internist—primary care doctor)
645 Washington St., Naperville, IL 60540; 630-525-8999

Jacob Jones, MD (Ophthalmologist)
UIC Eye Center, 1855 W. Taylor, Chicago, IL 60612-7243;
312-996-7030

Selden Berzynski, MD (Gastroenterologist)
645 S. Washington St., Naperville, IL 60540; 630-525-1235

DENTIST

David Denture, DDS
1842 Bay Swirl Court, Naperville, IL 60540; 630-727-1234

DRUG ALLERGIES: Penicillin, Sulfa

MEDICATIONS: Timolol 1 gtt OD qhs

ASA 325 mg qhs

Multi Vit 1 tab qhs

Hydrochlorthiazide 50 mg qam

HEALTH HISTORY

PROBLEM	STATUS/PROCEDURES	LAST EXAM
Hypertension	active	5/06/07
Glaucoma	active	8/12/06
	Bilat trabeculectomy 1997 Jacob Jones, MD	

Colonic Polyps	active	11/4/06

Polypectomy, 3/14/97, (Dx: benign adenoma)

Colonoscopy, 6/99, no polyps seen

Polypectomy, 11/4/03, (Dx: benign tubular adenoma)

Actinic Keratosis	active RX imiquimod x 12 wks 2005
Knee	inactive

Medial meniscectomy, 1975, A. Juliano, MD and 1979, Larry Johnson, MD

Inguinal Hernia	inactive

Inguinal heriorrhaphy, 1985, Philo Smitt, MD

Gilberts Syndrome	(benign hyperbilirubinemia)

VACCINATION RECORD

VACCINE	PRIMARY SERIES	LAST BOOSTER
DPT	childhood	2005
Polio	childhood	
Chicken Pox	disease	
MMR	disease X 3	
Smallpox	childhood	
Pneumovax	1978	2004
Influenza	annually	2004
Hepatitis B	3 doses heptavax	1986
TB tine test	2007 negative	

continues

continued

TESTS AND STUDIES

TEST / STUDY (most recent)				DATE
H pylori+ Rxed triple abx & Prilosec				7/20/93
EKG: Rate 47 Sinus Bradycardia (normal resting heart rate)				4/5/02
PSA:	0.8			6/21/99
PSA:	0.62			5/1/03
Homocysteine:	10.1			4/14/00
Cholesterol Total:	183 HDL 66 Trigl 120			5/1/07
CBC	WBC 6.5	HGB 14.7	HCT 41.5	5/1/07
GLUCOSE:	94			5/1/07
BUN: 14 CR	1.3			5/1/07
CA:	9.4			5/1/07
TBILI:	1.6			5/1/07
LFTs	normal			5/1/07
ELECTROLYTES	normal			5/1/07
BP	118/68			5/1/07
CARDIAC stress test bruce 7 (19'45") normal				1/5/05
	Resting pulse 48 EF 76% BP118/68			
	Max pulse 185 EF 90+% BP 160/80			
EKG NSR	normal see tracing (image)			5/1/07
CXR	Normal (image)			5/1/07

A list of previous hospitalizations, including hospital name, address, and date is important, too.

If you list all this information, you will have a better electronic medical record than just about anyone, including your doctor and hospital. In fact, encourage them to keep a copy.

Most people persist in thinking that "the doctor or the hospital has all my medical records." In some cases your doctor may be keeping very good records. But many people, especially those who are uninsured or have changed doctors, have incomplete, woefully inadequate records. This can be very dangerous in an emergency if you are unable to speak for yourself (and the medical records department is closed or otherwise unavailable) or cannot remember. An inadequate record can be very costly if it results in an unnecessary test or hospitalization (if, for example, you cannot produce a copy of your chronically abnormal EKG).

Now, believe it or not, you may also need financial information. For instance, if you are applying for insurance through the state, you will need to show your salary history as well as your previous insurance records. So, have all your financial records up-to-date, too, before you start applying for various policies.

> **Code Red**
>
> We cannot emphasize enough the importance of photocopies as well as computer records for your health, financial, and insurance information. And do not assume that if you send information to an insurance company or health provider once that you won't need to send it again. When Winnie, a writer, applied for insurance through the state, she had to send all of her records three times before the state considered her file complete.

Special Employment Situations

Because the majority of people in the United States who have insurance carry it through their employer, you will also have to provide your employment information to almost anyone you deal with in your quest for either medical care or public insurance.

For example, let's say you apply for a state-run program that helps women and children who survive on an amount of money within 300 percent of the Federal poverty level. The program administrators may want to know how you earn your money (i.e., what job you have and if you can verify that job with pay stubs) as well as whether your job offers health insurance. And, if it does, why aren't you accepting it?

The idea of sharing your pay stubs and your insurance options with someone might be scary, because you might feel like, on paper, it looks like you should be able to get insurance or health care. The reality, though, is that many administrators (both in health care and insurance) realize the discrepancy between how the situation looks on paper and how it actually plays out in real life.

For example, let's say you have a job as a barista at your local coffee chain. According to a popular coffee chain's union website:

> "... unless you are a shift supervisor, you will end up averaging less than 20 hours per week (and thus you will not be eligible for benefits). You might get 24 hours for a few weeks, then 16.5, then 12.25, then 15.25, then 20, then 16, then 12, then 8.75.

> "Even worse, you might initially average 20 hours per week, and you will get an enrollment form (for health benefits) in the mail. Then, your hours will start getting cut so that you are not eligible for benefits."

Furthermore, let's do the math. The average barista earns $7.00, so if she works 20 hours each week, she's earning $140. Imagine, then, how she's going to pay for health insurance. Let's say she's fortunate enough to earn the average wage of a major discount department store worker ($11.00 per hour) and work 40 hours per week. She's still only earning $440 each week. But those numbers are uncommonly generous.

def•i•ni•tion

Health Affairs, a medical publication, estimates that 16 million adults (above and beyond the 47 million uninsured) are **underinsured**, which means their insurance would not protect them against extremely high or catastrophic health care expenses.

Many times people who are employed part-time (or even almost full-time) in the service industry are often *underinsured*. In other words, their insurance helps them get some medical care, such as well visits or regular check-ups, but it would not help them in case of an emergency.

If you are underinsured and you want to apply for insurance coverage to protect you in case of an accident or serious illness, you will need records to show the insurance companies.

In fact, if you go online, you can find websites dedicated to the issues faced by employees of popular retail stores because they can't get enough hours to qualify for health coverage. This is a problem for any-one in retail, where low wages and high employee turnover makes it a very high expense for employers to offer great benefits. We point this out because we want to explain the difficulties part-time workers have when they try to get health care.

If you are a part-time worker, a retail worker, or someone who can't afford insurance premiums due to low hours or low wages, you can turn to your state insurance board to see if you qualify for subsidized health care or insurance. See Chapter 2 for more information on those programs. You can also purchase high-deductible insurance in case of emergency or catastrophic illness but pay for your own well visits and other preventive care out of your pocket. This kind of insurance is expensive, of course, but it may be less expensive than an insurance plan.

Another option is to band together with your co-workers, as the work-ers at Starbucks and Wal-Mart have done, to petition your company to grant you access to health care.

How to Be an Advocate

Remember the scene in the movie *Terms of Endearment* when Shirley MacLaine screams at the nurse to get her daughter pain medication? That's *advocacy*. Of course, you don't have to be a hysterical mother to be an advocate. You can be rational and forward thinking and simply help someone navi-gate bureaucracy to get the care he needs. Working to protect the rights of and to help take care of someone else is called *advocacy*.

def•i•ni•tion

Advocacy is to speak in sup-port or in favor of something. You can advocate in favor of a patient's health-care rights or health insurance rights in order to get him better care and financial protection.

Throughout this book, we talk about the numerous programs that are in place to help individuals who need it. If one program doesn't help, another usually will. Or a specific doctor will help. The problem, as we've said, is finding the time and energy to ask questions and tell people what you need.

That's where advocacy comes in. Sometimes advocacy simply means making phone calls or doing a web search for someone who doesn't have a computer. Most people who need help need money, of course, but they also need information. And when you are scared and sick, it is difficult to find the inner resources to stand up for yourself or to get the help you need.

Health care is not just an individual issue, but one that involves families and friends. We are aware that you might be reading this book because you are worried about the care of your child, parent, or a close friend.

> ### Bet You Didn't Know
>
> According to HIPAA (Health Insurance Portability and Accountability Act), a federal law, you have the right to all of your medical records. At the same time, doctors, hospitals, and insurance companies may not share your records without your permission. You give your permission for this to the insurance company when they write your policy.

Of course, if you go to the hospital or doctor's office with a friend or your parent, then the patient can simply tell the provider what information he can share. In fact, patients often benefit when they have someone with them because they are often scared or too confused to hear all of the medical information they are being given to make well-informed decisions.

Nevertheless, most health-care providers are very familiar with HIPAA regulations, so if you begin to make inquiring phone calls or ask a lot of questions seemingly without the patient's permission, the physician may request written permission for this type of communication.

First, get a signed, dated letter of authorization. Many states have specific health-care proxy forms for these situations. In a pinch, a verbal okay by the patient in the presence of the provider is usually enough. For telephone, e-mail, or regular mail contacts, you will probably need the signed form. If you are calling an insurance company or provider, simply telling the clerk that you are the person who pays the bill and identifying your legal relationship, such as spouse, parent, or adult child of an elderly parent, is often enough to at least speak to someone about payment if not about medical care. However, if you are a domestic partner, significant other, friend, or neighbor, you better have signed paperwork to show your legal rights to the information.

Next, learn as much as possible about the patient's history and medical condition. Physicians typically appreciate useful information from relatives about a patient's condition. Also, the more you know about the patient's history and medical condition, the better prepared you are to understand the options and treatment plans the doctor describes.

For Your Health

Most physicians are grateful when patients or patient advocates do research on the Internet, as long as they use reliable, accurate sources, such as the National Library of Medicine, The Mayo Clinic, or the *New England Journal of Medicine*.

If the person you are caring for is seriously ill, consider finding a medical professional, such as a doctor or nurse or a "professional patient advocate" to advocate for you or your loved one.

While in an ideal world, your primary care physician (PCP) would act as your advocate, he may or may not fully understand your personal, cultural, or religious situation or needs. He may have other conflicting priorities (such as other patients, time, or economic considerations) that limit his ability to fully advocate for his patient.

Your Spouse

In most cases, spouses have the right to make decisions for each other in medical emergencies. For example, according to the mental health laws in Louisiana, "a person suffering from substance abuse may be admitted and detained at a public or private general hospital or a substance abuse in-patient facility for observation, diagnosis, and treatment for a period not to exceed twenty-eight days, when a parent, spouse, or the major child of the person if that child has attained the age of 18 years has admitted the person or caused him to be admitted ..." but to do this, "the person, the parent, spouse, or the major child of the person if that child has attained the age of 18 years shall execute or provide a written statement of facts, including personal observations, leading to the conclusion that the person is suffering from substance abuse and is dangerous to himself or others or is gravely disabled, specifically describing any dangerous acts or threats, and stating that the person has been encouraged to seek treatment but is unwilling to be evaluated on a voluntary basis."

Nevertheless, also according to the law, "As soon as practicable, but in no event more than twelve hours after admission to the hospital or inpatient facility, a physician shall examine the person and either execute an emergency certificate … or order the person discharged."

In other words, a spouse can't simply be in control of a partner's health care without verifying, through written statement and via a third party, the reality of the situation.

Of course, as an individual you are not expected to know all of the laws that apply to you and your spouse, but your doctor, clinic, or emergency room will be very clear about the rights of each of you.

Your Parent

It is common knowledge that, as the baby boomers get older, more and more of them are finding themselves responsible for aging parents, even when those parents live far away.

If time allows, the first thing you and your parent need to do is sign a legal document (Health-care Power of Attorney) saying that you have permission to be a part of your parent's health decisions and health information. In this way, especially if you live far from your parent, you can be privy to their information and be able to help them.

Numerous organizations help adult caregivers for family members, including Eldercare (a government agency) at 1-800-677-1116 or www.eldercare.gov; Family Caregiver Alliance/National Center on Caregiving at 1-800-445-8106 or caregiver.org; and the National Alliance for Caregiving at caregiving.org.

For the most part, when you are dealing with issues relating to older people, you must familiarize yourself with Medicare as well as pensions.

For Your Health

If your parent has an attorney, the two of you can visit her to find out more about getting legal permission to share all medical information between you and the doctor. If you need to find a lawyer who specializes in this care, contact the National Academy of Elder Law Attorneys at 520-881-4005 or www.naela.org. This organization offers referrals to attorneys who specialize in law relating to aging and caregiving.

Domestic Partners

Just like all benefits to any individual, the type and usefulness of health-care insurance varies depending on the employer and the locality. Domestic partner benefits may include long-term care, group life insurance, family and bereavement leave, and most commonly, health, dental, and vision insurance.

Even more so, the definition of "domestic partner" varies from employer to employer. Some companies include same-sex couples, unmarried opposite-sex couples, and common law marriages. Others cover only same-sex partners on the grounds that opposite-sex couples can receive spousal benefits by getting married while same-sex couples do not have this option. Regardless of how the term is defined, employers typically require domestic partners to sign an affidavit stating that they are in a lasting, committed relationship. They may also require that a couple live together for a specified period of time before they become eligible for domestic partner benefits.

And with these rights sometimes come the rights of a divorcing spouse to ask that the covered spouse continue to carry health insurance for the family, despite the change in marital status.

Gay and Lesbian Relationships

As anyone who follows the news regarding domestic partners and other issues related to marriage and gay marriage rights knows, couples of all kinds have varying rights and responsibilities depending on the state in which they live, their status as a couple, and, in many cases, the company for which one of them works. In fact, it's harder to generalize about the situation of all couples than about nearly any other category of people in this book.

That's because more and more married heterosexual couples also have to make hard choices when it comes to health care and health insurance. Or, in the most likely scenario, one person in a couple will stay in a job or have a job that allows them to have good health benefits.

If you are gay or lesbian and single, then your sexual orientation may not necessarily matter when it comes to your health insurance. It may be more important to consider your financial and health status. However, if you are part of a couple, then you may prefer to buy health insurance that recognizes your status and orientation.

As a first step, ask friends or people who work at the local chapter of any gay, lesbian, bisexual, and transgender organizations to see if they know of GLBT-friendly insurers. Or, go to www. gayandlesbianinsuranceservices.com for more options.

Widow Rights

Each year in the United States about 800,000 people are widowed. These aren't always elderly people, of course, and the spouse who is left behind will be alone for approximately 14 years, according to Census statistics.

Since it's quite typical for one person in a family to carry the family's health insurance, the death of that person is not only emotionally upsetting but also financially difficult. Obviously many issues come up when someone dies, but when it comes to health insurance, it's important to know that the laws that cover dependents (including spouses) can fall under state or federal jurisdiction.

If the spouse who died covered the family with insurance he received through his employer, then, under federal law, dependents (like recently unemployed people) can decide to use COBRA (the Consolidated Omnibus Budget Reconciliation Act). This means a widow and any children or dependents can continue their current health insurance coverage for up to 36 months. COBRA isn't free, however (see Chapter 1). COBRA premiums can reach up to 102 percent of the employer's cost, but are usually around $1,100 a month for one family. COBRA only applies to companies with 20 or more employees.

For Your Health

If you are truly indigent or worried that you will be, call your local Medicaid office to see if you qualify. Go to www.cms.hhs.gov or call information to get the number of your state health department.

It's also possible that you and your children can get access to health insurance through the Health Insurance Portability and Accountability Act or HIPPA. But make sure your current insurance doesn't lapse and attempt to buy private insurance using this law within 62 days of being offered. This option, too, may not be affordable.

Your other option (assuming you can't get insurance through your own job) is to buy private insurance. But that is highly expensive. If money is an issue, about 43 states have plans that serve families with children whose income is too high for Medicaid but too low for private premium payments (see Chapter 2 as well as Chapter 6 about health care for children).

College Students and Recent Grads

Even when they are employed, young people are more likely to have jobs that don't include health insurance as part of the benefits package. And even if an employer claims to offer insurance, they often only offer it to full-time employees, and most of the largest employers are clever about finding ways to minimize an employee's work hours, making them, in effect, ineligible for coverage. This situation is especially easy to exploit in retail jobs.

Bet You Didn't Know

A 2003 study found that young adults between the ages of 19 and 29 are the fastest-growing segment of the uninsured market. In 2005, nearly 30 percent of people between the ages of 19 and 24 lacked health insurance, ten percent higher than those 10 to 20 years older.

And if you're on the younger end of that range, there's a good chance you think you don't need insurance, unless of course, you have a disease or have been in an accident, in which case you might be desperate to get insurance.

In fact, young nonimmigrants are the largest group of people in the United States who are most likely not to have health insurance for several reasons.

Healthcare and Health Insurance Advocacy in General

Anyone can be an advocate for change. You can advocate for small changes, such as coverage for certain procedures or care within one insurance company's plan. Or you can advocate for large changes, such as the complete overhaul of medical insurance in the United States.

We would not presume to tell you which issues you might want to advocate for, of course, but we can give you some basic advocacy rules to use whether you are trying to make sure your child is covered for a cochlear implant or you are writing to your Congressperson regarding the inequities of the entire health insurance system.

By the way, these guidelines are in no specific order, but you need to have all of them in place to make your case.

- ◆ Be specific
- ◆ Talk or write to the correct person
- ◆ Be persistent
- ◆ Back up your claims
- ◆ Ask others to join you

The health insurance and health-care industry in the United States is certainly a subject that provokes anger in many people (especially those without insurance). If you are in a situation you would like to change, take action. As we mentioned earlier in this book, somewhere around 47 million Americans don't have insurance, so you certainly aren't alone.

The Least You Need to Know

◆ Finding insurance and health care requires much legwork and paperwork. You need—at the very least—your social security number, medical history, insurance records, and this same information for anyone who might be on your policy.

◆ Every state has specific regulations regarding the health care and health insurance rights for domestic partners, GLBT couples, widows, and college students.

◆ Being an advocate means speaking out for the rights of someone. You can help others get health coverage and health care, but always have written permission if you do this for anyone other than your child.

◆ Always keep your own medical records, especially if you change physicians or do not have health insurance. Do not assume that a doctor or hospital has your complete records or that your paperwork is available to consultants or other professionals.

Chapter 4

Creating Your Own Health Insurance Plan

In This Chapter

- Is cash still king?
- Walk-in clinics at your local drugstore
- Deductible details
- HSAs, FSAs, and other tax plans
- Medications and prescriptions

According to the National Coalition on Health Care, a non-partisan group that counts former Presidents George H. W. Bush and Jimmy Carter as honorary co-chairs, the "health care system is riddled with inefficiencies, excessive administrative expenses, inflated prices, poor management, and inappropriate care, waste and fraud. These problems significantly increase the cost of medical care and health insurance for employers and workers and affect the security of families."

With all of these paperwork problems, it's surprising that so many Americans think having insurance is the solution to getting better health care. It would seem the more useful way to take care of yourself is not to spend your energy getting insurance but, instead, to spend your energy (and money) getting medical care and dealing directly with doctors on a cash basis.

But is this possible? Is it possible to simply pay for health care as you need it? Well, yes and no. It's not as simple as it sounds for a couple of reasons. First, you need to have cash since many doctors will not see you if they don't know how you will pay them. Second, you need to be aware that if you get hurt or sick, your medical bills can end up being astronomical, i.e., more money than almost any citizen can afford on her own. Third, in Massachusetts at least (and soon probably in some other states), you have to have health insurance. It's the law.

Nevertheless, since the health insurance system is broken you might want to look at ways in which you can opt out of the system and still stay healthy. Or at least find out how you might manage the system rather than having the system manage you.

Will Your Doctor Take Cash?

Remember cash? Before the age of managed care health plans, when someone was sick or wanted a check-up, she made an appointment with a doctor and then paid the bill. If she was able to get reimbursed from an insurance company, she simply sent in the bill to them and waited for a check.

Well, guess what? You can still do this. There are doctors among us who work outside of the insurance system. Most doctors, clinics, or hospitals will happily accept cash. Here's how to find them: dial the phone.

All you need to do is ask. Call the doctor, and ask if she will accept payment at the time of the appointment.

Of course, there are a couple of issues here. Maybe you don't have the money to pay for an appointment. Second, your visit to the doctor may be the first step in your health care so you know that further down the road more bills and expenses will await you. But that doesn't mean you shouldn't try this option.

High deductible indemnity insurance (for emergencies) coupled with a Health Savings Account for regular doctor visits is a good way to facilitate dealing with your physician on a cash basis and put the patient (not the insurance company) back in control of her healthcare.

For Your Health

According to a study published in the New England Journal of Medicine (July 2007), when a patient's doctors work together coordinating care, they can often keep their patients out of the hospital and reduce overall health care spending. If you have more than one regular doctor, have them stay in touch with each other about your health and their treatment.

It is the responsibility of your primary care doctor, usually a family practitioner, internist, or pediatrician, to coordinate care with your specialists. Let your doctor know that you expect him to do this and appreciate his efforts. In order to insure that this occurs, become the messenger and carry records, reports, and test results back to your PCP from consultants. Mention to the consultant that you want your PCP to receive a copy of his report. Bottom line, in our current fractured system, you have the ultimate responsibility to make this happen.

Negotiating Price with a Doctor

Well, you know the obvious information you will need to give a doctor: name, address, social security number, phone, and emergency contact information, not to mention allergies and the reason for your visit. But, of course, you know what the doctor really wants to know: who is paying for the visit?

The answer to this question will depend on your circumstances and, of course, the physician will appreciate your honest answers. It will help you, too, to know if this is a physician who will care for a patient without insurance.

- ◆ If you have just lost your insurance but have seen the doctor before and have a specific reason for wanting to see him again, when you call to make an appointment, tell the nurse that you no longer have insurance, and ask what the doctor would charge you for a noninsured visit. Very likely, a doctor who knows you will offer you a reduced rate for a cash payment.

◆ If you cannot pay the full amount for your visit, explain how much you can pay or how much you can pay in installments. On the assumption that you like this doctor and she likes you, it is possible that this will work for your next visit (although possibly not as a way to get ongoing care).

◆ If you cannot pay at all, tell the nurse or doctor your problem, your financial situation, and that you are looking into getting public medical assistance. Ask the doctor's receptionist if she can help you get coverage and if the doctor can see you before the paperwork has gone through.

◆ If you went to see the doctor without previously telling him that you no longer have insurance, then you may end up feeling awkward in the waiting room when the nurse asks if you are still covered by Insurer XYZ. Now, it's possible, if you have just lost your insurance (i.e., in the past week or two) that you can still give them your card and, if they call to verify, your records won't have changed. You can take that chance. However, you should know that you are responsible for payment—not the insurer—so if the insurer refuses to pay the bill, the doctor will then bill you.

If you want to keep seeing this doctor, then be honest about your situation. Let's face it—if there are 47 million uninsured Americans, chances are he has other patients who are in this situation. And most doctors have the same problems with the health insurance industry that you do, so they will work with you, not against you, to try to take care of you and get you covered for the cost of their care.

If your doctor doesn't want to buck the system or doesn't want to treat you—with or without insurance—he is within his rights not to serve you. He is supposed to help you find another physician (especially if you live somewhere with few health care options or if you have a condition that requires specialized treatment or knowledge), but a doctor doesn't have to take care of whoever walks in his door, unless your life is in danger. And then, all he is required to do is his best to make sure you don't die—which might include simply calling an ambulance.

Remember doctors need to get paid for their work. Even if you have a negative opinion of how well they are paid, that shouldn't be part of your negotiation as that won't help you communicate with your doctor, nor is it the point.

Now the preceding list will help you if you are seeing a doctor you know and who knows you. If you do not have health insurance and want to see a new doctor who has a private practice (i.e., who doesn't work in a clinic or walk-in facility), you should also tell them your financial situation ahead of time. And be sure to bring all of your medical records. If the physician has a dedicated insurance worker on staff, then she may be able to help you with your coverage and payment issues.

Drugstores and supermarkets now sometimes have walk-in clinics right past the checkout counters. If you don't have a doctor or insurance, it might be best to just go to one of these when you are sick. Many of them are chains, and most are less expensive than a private doctor. If you want to find one, look in the phone book or call a local hospital. They sometimes have clinics on site.

This is a relatively new phenomenon, a direct outgrowth of chain retailers' optical and pharmacy operations. These clinics are mostly staffed by nurse practitioners under the supervision of a doctor, who may be supervising numerous clinics and not physically present. They are economical places to get routine vaccinations, physical exams, and care for relatively minor illnesses, which is what they are primarily designed to do.

It is most important that you feel that practitioners at these clinics have the good clinical sense to make appropriate referrals when there are serious issues. In terms of when and if to utilize them, common sense should prevail.

At the present time there are numerous initiatives with the goal of nothing less than "revolutionizing" health care.

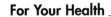

For Your Health

Steve Case's new company, Revolution Health, aims to put your health care in your hands. His site, www.revolutionhealth. com, has reliable health information, health insurance information, as well as telephone services so you can speak to an expert in either of these fields (for a membership fee of $129 each year).

At the risk of my reputation as a futurist, I predict that any significant advances in the delivery of health care in the United States and the world will spring from these initiatives, rather than any politically mandated system. If the study of history allows us to predict the future, then I am on sound footing with this opinion.

Some of the same minds and talent who brought us the computer revolution, and not a few doctors and Wall Street types are intensely focused on this market.

Creating Your Own Health Insurance Plan

When Carrie, a personal trainer and single mother, lost her job and insurance, she couldn't afford COBRA payments, so she bought private insurance. For one year, at a time when she earned about $35,000 annually, she paid $6,000 to insure herself and her son. They went to the doctor twice during that time, for well visits. And what was the total cost of those visits, had they paid cash? About $300.

Now of course, Carrie and her son were lucky; they were both in excellent health. But she really could have used that $6,000. A couple of times she used a credit card check to pay her rent because she was so short on cash, so really, the insurance contributed to a further problem with money.

People make choices like these all the time: health care or rent? Health care or food?

Meanwhile, Carrie's friend, Bob, was a contractor. He ran his own one-man business and didn't bother to carry health insurance even though one could argue that he's in a risky profession, being on construction sites and all. Instead, he put some money into an account each month—aside from his regular savings—to use for doctor visits and any other health care. Would the money in this account have covered him in case of emergency? No. But did he year after year save himself money? Absolutely.

So, here's the idea behind your own personal health insurance savings plan: put your own money in an interest-bearing account and save it. Use it for doctor visits, co-pays, medication, dental care, eyeglasses, and so on. If you are employed, you may be able to get a tax deduction on most of this through a Flex spending account. If you are unemployed/underemployed, you probably aren't paying (much) taxes. Build a nest egg over time, and earmark it for medical care. If you don't spend it all by age 65, you may have accumulated a significant amount.

The most cost-effective health insurance plan is one where you pay all the up front costs yourself and have catastrophic high deductible coverage for serious illness. This assumes you are relatively healthy and can afford the out-of-pocket costs of routine care. First dollar coverage (what everyone wants) is *very expensive*, and the premiums alone may kill you or your employer. The money saved on premiums with a high-deductible policy should be set aside to pay for preventive care, routine visits, and episodic care.

Low Versus High Deductibles

One of the terms you will hear a lot as you investigate buying insurance is deductible. A *deductible* is a specific amount you need to pay before an insurance company will begin to pay toward your claim.

Many people without employer-sponsored health insurance look into buying plans that will at least allow them to be covered in case of disaster. These plans, which are sometimes called catastrophic or high-deductible plans, kick in once someone has paid a higher amount of money than he would

def•i•ni•tion

A **deductible** is an agreed amount an insured person making a claim against an insurance policy must pay before an insurer will pay any compensation.

have had to pay with a lower-deductible plan. You don't have to pay a lot for them on a regular basis because the insurance company is betting that you won't get a serious illness or be in an accident.

High-deductible plans are often good for young adults who only see a doctor once or twice a year, but they are not right for everyone.

When you get a diagnosis of a life-threatening illness, you want to find the doctors and hospitals that can provide the best possible care. Not only do you want the right treatment, provided by a medical expert in whom you can feel confident, but you also want a doctor who treats you with respect, listens to your questions and concerns, and responds to them in an appropriate and timely manner.

Itemize on Your Taxes

Many medical expenses are tax-deductible, but to take these deductions, you need to file something other than the 1040 or 1040EZ because you need to itemize. So of course, save all your receipts, including those from office visits, prescriptions, and any lab or other tests.

Most patients who get their insurance from their employers are able to invest in Flexible Spending Accounts (FSAs). This plan allows workers to take money out of their paycheck, before they pay taxes on that income, to use exclusively for health-care expenses. Likewise, many employees pay their health insurance premiums with pretax dollars, which means not only are they getting some of their health insurance paid for by an employer, but they are also getting a discount on their own contributions.

> **Bet You Didn't Know**
>
> Personal insurance premiums are not tax deductible, unless they exceed 7.5 percent of your income. However, if you are self-employed or can open a flexible spending account, you can get different tax breaks to cover the premiums. They are tax-deductible for an employer.

All of these ways to save are completely unfair to the person who chooses not to chain himself to a large corporation. But that doesn't mean you are completely out of luck if you don't have employer-sponsored insurance. And by the way, while the paperwork is a real pain in the neck, so is sitting at a desk in a job you don't like just so you can get insurance.

But, you can get tax deductions without itemizing—by using Health Savings Accounts.

Health Savings Accounts

A Health Savings Account (HSA) is a *tax-sheltered* savings account earmarked for medical expenses. Deposits made to an HSA are 100 percent tax-deductible for the self-employed as well as others who open HSAs. You simply withdraw the money by check or debit card when you need to pay low-cost medical bills, such as check-ups and well visits, prescription costs, and more inexpensive tests.

You cannot use the money in an HSA for higher-cost medical expenses because you can't deposit that much money into an HSA account; there are limits. Therefore, you need to also carry health insurance for catastrophic or high cost events. Nevertheless, the money in the account accrues interest, and if you don't use it all, you can keep it indefinitely, even until you retire.

def•i•ni•tion

When a financial account is **tax-sheltered,** the money isn't taxed by the Internal Revenue Service. Therefore, it is an extra savings to you. Once you put the money into an HSA or other tax shelter, you can't claim the deduction on your income taxes since you've already taken the deduction.

HSAs are meant to replace traditional health insurance policies that include low co-pays but also come with many restrictions. When you use a health savings plan you have a higher degree of freedom regarding your choice of doctors, which typically comes from a PPO directory, without the extensive restrictions imposed by HMO-type plans. It also provides you the ability to pay cash with all its attendant advantages.

And more and more Americans are signing up for HSAs. According to the America Health Insurance Providers (AHIP), in 2004 about 438,000 individuals were covered by HSA-type insurance plans, while in 2005 3.2 million people were covered. And those Americans are investing about $1 billion in these accounts, according to Inside Consumer-Directed Care (ICDC).

Anyone over the age of 18 can contribute to an HSA if he:

◆ Has coverage under an HSA-qualified "high deductible health plan" (HDHP)

◆ Has no other "first-dollar" medical coverage. "First dollar" coverage means plans such as Medicare, Tricare, Flexible Spending Arrangements, and Health Reimbursement Arrangements. You can have other types of insurance, such as specific injury insurance or accident, disability, dental care, vision care, or long-term care insurance.

◆ Is not enrolled in Medicare.

◆ Cannot be claimed as a dependent on someone else's tax return.

There is no income limit on who can establish an HSA, and you, your employer, or both of you can contribute to this account, which is especially good if you work for a small employer who can't carry a full insurance plan for you and other employees. If you have regular medical expenses that you would like to reduce through a tax deduction, you can always ask your employer to contribute in lieu of a raise or as an additional benefit.

Code Red

Although, in the words of the Treasury Department, there are no "use it or lose it rules" on HSAs, if your employer contributes, he is entitled to some of the money, too. Make sure you, he, and the bank or an accountant can explain to both of you what your responsibilities and benefits are. While any unspent balances in your account stay in your individual account, if the account belongs to you and your employer, he may be entitled to some of the money if you leave the company.

In 2007, the maximum amount that a person can contribute (and deduct) to an HSA from all sources is $2,850 for an individual or $5,650 for a family. If you are over 55, you are allowed to make additional "catch-up" contributions to your health savings accounts. In 2007, 55+ people can add $800; for 2008 it is $900; and for 2009 and after, you may contribute an additional $1,000 a year.

You control your HSA completely, which includes deciding:

◆ Where you deposit the money. You can use a bank, credit union, or an insurance company. The government says this about it: "Entities already approved by the IRS to be an IRA or an Archer MSA trustee or custodian. Other entities can apply to the IRS to be approved as a non-bank trustee or custodian." You can call your bank or credit union to ask if they are approved for HSAs, or go online to www.hsainsider.org and input your zip code to find approved entities.

◆ What kind of account you want it to be. You can choose any type of savings plan. So as well as choosing the bank, you can also open an account with lower management fees, higher interest rates, a variety of investment options, or more security, such as whether the account is FDIC insured.

◆ When and how much you want to contribute. The more you contribute, the greater your tax savings, but if money is tight or you want to make one large contribution rather than a few small ones, you can do that. So, there is no timetable as to when you make your deposits unless you choose an account with automatic deductions or another type of deposit policy.

◆ How much you want to use for medical expenses. This is your money you are spending for medical care. Thus, the HSA creates an incentive for you, as the holder, to be a wise consumer of medical care. You may be more inclined to spend your money on preventive measures, such as flu vaccines, rather than on more expensive treatments.

◆ Which medical expenses you want to pay from the account. However, all of the expenses have to be "qualified medical expenses" (see "What is a 'Qualified Medical Expense?'" later in the chapter) according to the IRS. And if you want, you can pay cash for some of your medical expenses and simply keep the money in your account for a rainy (or unhealthy) day.

Here's an example: let's say you have $1,400 in your HSA and you decide to get a flu shot that costs $35.00. You have $35.00 in your wallet, so you don't have to take the money out of your account. Instead, you can just keep the $35.00 in savings and let it continue to collect interest or just be there for you. This is especially helpful if you are a freelancer and aren't always sure about your income. Likewise, sometimes those expenses aren't $35.00, but a few hundred dollars, so it's good to do the savings when you can.

Catastrophic Insurance

This policy will cover you for the high-dollar expenses, which usually occur suddenly. What if you or your child is diagnosed with cancer? Or what if you get struck by a hit-and-run driver? It would be bad enough to be sick—you don't want to add bankruptcy to your injuries! Often this type of situation is really why we want health insurance. And the insurance available for these types of emergencies is called catastrophic insurance or high-deductible coverage.

Catastrophes are expensive. But having a policy that covers catastrophes means that you will have to pay all the costs short of a catastrophe, thus the high deductible on these insurance policies. The HSA lets you pay those deductible expenses with tax-sheltered dollars.

If you are going to invest in catastrophic health insurance or a High Deductible Health Plan (HDHP), do it in conjunction with an HSA. What are the requirements? They vary by the year, but for 2007, the catastrophic health insurance plan must have a minimum deductible of $1,100 for an individual and $2,200 for a family. Annual out-of-pocket expenses, including co-pays and deductibles, cannot exceed $5,500 for an individual and $11,000 for a family. These amounts will be indexed annually for inflation.

Bet You Didn't Know

Insurance makes a difference in your health; so while you can still get health care without it (and this entire book is dedicated to helping you do that) we want to tell you that you should always be open, if money allows or if you qualify for public insurance, to getting insurance, because, according to the Kaiser Commission on Medicaid and the Uninsured (2002), the uninsured have a 10 to 15 percent higher mortality rate and earn 10 to 30 percent less because of their poor health.

The Health Coverage Tax Credit

In 2002, Congress enacted The Health Coverage Tax Credit (HCTC) as part of the Trade Act, specifically for manufacturing workers who lose health insurance as a result of foreign competition. The credit, which is equal to 65 percent of the premium for qualified coverage, is also available to some early retirees who lost pension benefits.

To qualify for the HCTC you must meet certain requirements, such as being enrolled in a qualified health plan. And, since it is a tax credit, you need to use an IRS Form (#8885) to claim the HCTC on your tax return. The credit is given to you when your premiums are due or when you file your federal tax return.

Talk to an accountant, as well as your state's health department, to find out if you qualify and how much coverage would cost (remember, you can only get the credit if you are paying for coverage). Note that no available state-qualified plans exist in Delaware, Hawaii, Mississippi, Nevada, New Mexico, Puerto Rico, South Dakota, and Wyoming.

Find a Group

One of the best ways to get insurance is to get group insurance (and thus group rates) through a professional or other type of organization. For example, if you're a writer, you can join AvantGuild, a group of freelance writers, editors, and other publishing types. Because so many people in this career work on their own as freelancers, they benefit by joining together and purchasing health insurance as a group. In this way, they get group rates without having to get a staff job.

If you are a professional, look into groups that include, with their membership, the chance to purchase health insurance. Other groups that often try to get group health insurance rates are alumni associations and fraternal organizations. And many of these groups have lots of other benefits, such as networking, the chance to do charity work, and the opportunity to take classes to forward your career.

Prescriptions

Take a guess. How much did Americans spend on *prescription drugs* in 2005, according to the Kaiser Family Foundation? 50 billion dollars? 100 billion dollars? If either of those numbers seem unbelievable to you, hang on. Americans spent over 200 billion dollars on prescription drugs in 2005.

def•i•ni•tion

> **Prescription drugs** are substances intended to diagnose, cure, treat, or prevent medical conditions or diseases. Before they can be legally marketed, these drugs must undergo clinical studies on their safety and effectiveness and be approved by the FDA. The agency approves a drug if its experts determine that the benefits of the drug outweigh the risks associated with it. But no drug is absolutely safe; some level of risk always exists.

This number is not surprising, of course, since some of the most prescribed medications, such as Prozac and Lipitor, are advertised directly to consumers on TV and in magazines.

While most employer-based insurance plans offer drug coverage, people with private insurance or no insurance often struggle to find ways to pay for medication they need. And even with low co-pays, noncompliance (i.e., not taking medications) is a problem for patients and business.

The Integrated Benefits Institute conducted a three-year study on patients with rheumatoid arthritis who had employer-sponsored prescription drug coverage and found that half the patients were not taking their drugs. These patients said they considered the out-of-pocket co-payments too high even though the co-payments averaged $26 for a 30-day supply. As a result, the institute's study found, the employers incurred $17.2 million in costs from lost productivity, 26 percent more than the estimate of what they would have spent if the workers had taken their arthritis drugs.

Because the issue of noncompliance, for financial and other reasons, is so large, even supermarkets are trying to help consumers with prescription drug cost. Publix, for example, in Florida and a few other Southern states, will offer seven of the most widely prescribed antibiotics at no cost. You must have a physician's prescription, but with one, you can receive 14-day supplies of amoxicillin, cephalexin, ciprofloxacin, penicillin VK, ampicillin, and erythromycin. And Kmart and Wal-Mart stores sell prescriptions at low cost.

More and more Americans are finding creative ways to get their medications, some more successful than others. Ordering over the Internet (who knows where the drugs are coming from and if their production is regulated so you know what you're getting?) and going to another country (some countries are more reliable than others about regulating drug production) are two options. And others just take their medicines sporadically, which can be dangerous to their health.

Even with coverage, medication costs can be more than burdensome for an average family. For example, James and Sue are a couple in their early 60s who live in New Jersey. James has long been a well-paid consultant in the computer industry, but as a consultant, he has no employer-based health insurance. He has a rare auto-immune based skin disease that is easily controlled by a medication. One pill a day is all he needs to take to stay completely healthy and symptom free. However, the pill costs $20 a day or $600 a month.

Sue, his wife, has a management position at a state university. While she loves her job, she is also ready to retire. However, because James cannot get any kind of insurance (health or life) due to this condition, she continues working solely to avoid the expense of paying for the medication out-of-pocket.

Is there a better way?

Why Is Medicine Different from Medical Care?

Unfortunately, there is no such thing as a "medicine" emergency. If you go to a hospital emergency room, you will be cared for, but while the doctor might be able to give you a few days' worth of medicine, neither he nor your local pharmacy can give you a complete prescription for free. Even most courses of antibiotics run for at least 10 days or two weeks, so what are you supposed to do if you need medicine and you don't have cash?

First, tell the doctor you don't have insurance—or you don't have prescription drug insurance. Lots of physicians, hospitals, and clinics have samples of drugs that pharmaceutical companies hand out. Most doctors are more than happy to offer them to sick patients who need them.

Also pharmaceutical manufacturers make their drugs available to low-income patients, as well as federally funded clinics at a discounted price. To learn more about these programs, call the pharmaceutical company who makes your specific medication or look on the company website for this information.

In 2005, the Pharmaceutical Research and Manufacturers of America began the Partnership for Prescription Assistance. These programs are not meant to be long-term sources of medication, but instead are to be used as a "last resort" for people who have exhausted all public program options, have no private insurance, and have low incomes.

> **Bet You Didn't Know**
>
> According to the National Health Policy Forum, pharmaceutical companies make available about $4 to $5 billion in drugs annually, equivalent to nearly 5 percent of total drug spending in the United States.

About 180 manufacturer-sponsored Prescription Assistance Programs, or PAPs, provide qualified low-income people with medications they couldn't otherwise purchase.

Medications can be very expensive even with insurance, so Volunteers in Health Care, which is based in the Brown University Center for Primary Care and Prevention, created RxAssist (www.rxassist.com), a pharmaceutical access information center funded by foundations, corporate sponsorships, and private donations. RxAssist maintains a database of PAPs as well as links and other information for patients who need help paying for their medications.

> **For Your Health**
>
> Not all drugs are available through Prescription Assistance Programs, but about 3,000 name-brand and generics are. To learn more go to www. needymeds.com.

Most manufacturer PAPs provide only brand-name drugs to their customers and only while the drug is protected by a patent. This is good because they are trying to help patients when the drug is most expensive.

On the other hand, sometimes it is possible to use less expensive generic drugs, which are often under $5 for a one-month supply. Because of generics, many large pharmacy retailers, such as Wal-Mart, Kmart, and Target, have created programs with guaranteed low prices for some generic drugs.

You may have to ask your physician to request the drug for you from the PAP. At the very least, you will be required to give your doctor's name and, often, her signature to apply to the PAP. If you need a high-cost or rare drug (a cancer drug, for example), ask if someone in your doctor's office has applied to these programs before.

> **For Your Health**
>
> Not all generic drugs are cheap. Some newly approved generics (which means one manufacturer has the generic patent after the original patent has ended) are priced at higher levels than more commonly used generics.

You will rarely get the drugs delivered to you. Instead, they will be sent to your doctor's office or straight to the pharmacy.

Can you see the potential problem? If you're looking for a short-term prescription, such as an antibiotic, you might be better off asking your doctor for samples rather than going through the rigmarole and waiting time of applying to a PAP program.

And another issue may make your doctor reluctant to help you apply—a lot of time and paperwork is involved in the process. Patients and physicians must prove no insurance program or money is available for the patient and the medication. It's a lot of work! If you want to apply, talk to your doctor about helping out

> **Code Red**
>
> Not taking your necessary medication because of cost can cause more health problems, which can land you in the hospital, thus resulting in medical bills. The most effective—and least expensive—thing you can do is take your medicine.

with the paperwork if you can. At the very least, show some appreciation for the hours her staff will put in to help you get your medication.

Bet You Didn't Know

Because of the costs and problems associated with the pharmaceutical industry, many states have programs in place to help its citizens obtain prescriptions. For example, in Virginia, the Rx Partnership makes free prescription drugs available to clinics and community health centers. The program distributed nearly $2 million in drugs in its first year of operation.

Illegal websites violate the rules of the FDA by selling prescription drugs without valid prescriptions. The FDA leaves it to states to decide what is a valid prescription. Websites cannot dispense drugs in violation of those laws or with no prescription at all. But they do it anyway.

Do not use sites that dispense drugs only after you fill out an online questionnaire as part of a consultation. Here's why: you can't be sure you are getting the right medication at all. You may just want to refill your Glucophage scrip, for example, but a site that doesn't require a valid prescription may not be conscientious enough to even send you a real medication.

The drugs you get (for a considerable amount of money) could be "outdated, contaminated, too potent or not potent enough, improperly manufactured and handled, or counterfeit," according to the NABP.

Code Red

To report a problem with a website selling medications, call 301-443-1240.

Problems with online prescriptions are common. In just six months, the NABP typically receives over 100 complaints related to medications online.

If you do want to buy medication online, make sure the site you are using is licensed by a state. Look for pharmacies that are extensions of traditional brick-and-mortar chain drug stores such as Walgreens, Eckerd, and CVS.

Remember legitimate sites require valid prescriptions, and if there is no way to contact the website pharmacy by phone or if prices are dramatically lower than the competition, then it's probably not a legitimate pharmacy.

Bet You Didn't Know

The FDA reports that approximately 200 domestic websites dispense prescription drugs without an online prescribing service. These are mostly American businesses, such as drugstore.com. You send in your prescription to buy a medication online. However, at least 400 websites dispense and prescribe medications, and half of these sites are located in foreign countries.

Why don't those sites selling unregulated medications get shut down? It's actually hard to find the source of many sites, which have multiple links. And, according to the FDA, there are jurisdictional challenges because "the regulatory and enforcement issues cross state, federal, and international lines."

Alternative Treatments

We didn't write this book to give you medical treatment advice, but we can tell you that many alternatives to Western medicines provide relief and cures to Western ailments. Massage, acupuncture, and other alternatives have been shown to be effective remedies for some illnesses.

And while many of these treatments aren't covered by insurance, the good news is that, without insurance, you are free to spend your medical dollars where you want. If your muscles ache, you can go to a sports medicine physician, or you can go to a massage therapist. You won't have to worry about getting a referral or making sure your massage therapist is in the network!

Once you do get insurance (if you do), more and more of these treatments are being covered by employer-sponsored policies.

In fact, 14 major HMOs and insurance providers, including Aetna, Medicare, Prudential, and Kaiser Permanente, cover some alternative therapies. Oxford Health Plans was the first major health care plan in this country to offer comprehensive coverage for a range of alternative care services, including acupuncture, chiropractic, naturopathy, nutrition, yoga, and massage therapy if policy holders paid an additional premium.

Code Red

Charlatans have preyed on the unsuspecting since time immemorial. It is especially distressing, however, in cases where effective (even life saving) medical treatments are foregone in favor of worthless potions, "products," or treatments. People with incurable, even fatal conditions often fall prey to pseudoscientific (usually expensive) therapies hawked on the Internet, in exotic locales, and by "alternative" practitioners.

Remember 40 percent of (real) pain will respond to placebo (sham) treatment. This is why controls are used for comparison in scientific studies. Many (minor) ailments will respond to a placebo based on the "power of positive thinking"—if you think it will work, it will.

Your primary care physician may be a good sounding board before indulging in some forms of "alternative care."

Insurers who offer some coverage of alternative and complementary medicines include American Western Life Insurance Company, Blue Cross/Blue Shield, Kaiser Permanente, Mutual of Omaha, Prudential, Tufts, and Harvard. Usually these plans cover chiropractic care— acupuncture, biofeedback, massage therapy, and some herbal remedies.

Bet You Didn't Know

In 1997 a National Institutes of Health panel found that acupuncture is effective in treating postoperative and chemotherapy nausea, vomiting, and other conditions. It has also been shown to be effective in pain management.

To learn more about what therapies might work for you and how to best pay for them, including insurance policies that allow alternative and complementary medicines, go to the National Center for Complementary and Alternative Medicine (part of the National Institutes of Health) at nccam.nih.gov. If you click on nccam.nih.gov/health/financial, you will learn more about paying for these treatments.

The Least You Need to Know

- ◆ Have an expert, such as an accountant, run the numbers about how you can best pay for your healthcare within your financial situation, taking into account all of the savings plans and account information.

◆ Be completely honest with doctors and other medical professionals about your financial and insurance situation. Do not assume that a doctor is on the side of the insurance company or doesn't sympathize with your situation.

◆ Contact pharmaceutical manufacturers to find out if they have programs to help offset the cost of medications for their customers.

◆ Call your state's insurance board to find out about public options and rules governing insurance plans and coverage.

◆ Alternative therapies should be approached with a healthy skepticism and with prior advice from your doctor. Be aware that not all health accounts will reimburse you for those expenses.

Part 2

Getting Care on an Ongoing Basis

You might not have healthcare coverage, but you still need health care. Whether you're having a baby, need treatment for a condition such as diabetes, or want a routine checkup (most conditions that kill Americans, such as heart disease and cancer, are detectable by physicians during routine visits), Part 2 has you covered. Don't skip Chapter 11 on elective surgery, either. You might be surprised to learn that elective surgery can include gallbladder removal, hysterectomies, hernia repairs, and other procedures.

Chapter 5

General Health Care

In This Chapter

- ◆ Finding a doctor and specialists
- ◆ Getting reliable health information
- ◆ Donating blood
- ◆ "Free" clinics
- ◆ Tests at local pharmacies/supermarkets

One of the reasons HMOs didn't work well for most patients was the lack of a personal connection between the patient and the doctor. In the 1980s and '90s, when someone went to a typical HMO, he saw whichever doctor was around, rather than one with whom he had established a relationship. Most of us want to feel like our doctor genuinely knows us and actually cares about our well-being. We don't want a doctor who seems to care only about his paycheck or who thinks of medicine as only a science and not a job that involves individuals who are often scared and vulnerable.

And of course, a patient feels more vulnerable when he doesn't have insurance or isn't financially secure. It is embarrassing and difficult to ask for help from someone in a position of power, like a doctor. Most of us want to walk into a doctor's office with the security that we will get the care we need and the freedom to pay for it without worrying about overwhelming bills.

Picking a Doctor and Specialist

Before we discuss how to find the right doctor and how to pay for your care, you should know that research has shown the quality of a doctor's care is not directly related to the fee he charges. According to Aetna, an insurance company that practices price transparency (i.e., patients know what each doctor and provider charges for a service and what the discount is to Aetna), there is little or no difference in the quality of care when price is compared. In other words, when it comes to medical care, you don't necessarily get what you pay for.

For Your Health

No matter what doctor you choose and how you pay for your care, if you are diagnosed with something serious that requires extensive and ongoing care, consider getting a second opinion. Even people with insurance often end up paying cash for second opinions as it is sometimes better to go out of a network or to a completely new doctor who you only see once to get the most detached point of view possible.

If you do go for a second opinion, be careful not to delay care for a potentially time-sensitive and serious problem. Also try to think ahead about what you will do if the second opinion is at odds with the first. Will you go for a third opinion and take the best two out of three, stick with the doctor who seems nicer, or try to persuade the doctor to do what you want to do, which isn't always a good idea since your emotions can cloud your judgment?

Finding a Doctor

Unless you are in an emergency situation, consider your first visit to a doctor to be similar to a job interview—and you are the potential boss or at least co-worker with power. You are interviewing the physician to experience how he treats his patients. Is he kind? Understanding? Impatient? Disorganized? Do you feel he is knowledgeable about health and, specifically, any problems you have, such as diabetes, heart disease, or mental health disorder? We know a woman who went to see a gyne-cologist about birth control and told the new doctor she had become severely depressed on the birth control pill and wanted another option. When the gynecologist began to tell her about new types of birth control pills, the woman realized she needed to find a different doctor just as much as she needed new medication.

Even without insurance, you should have a primary care physician (PCP). Your PCP may be able to help you with specialty referrals (and figuring out which specialist to see), admission to the hospital, and coordinating care for you over the years. Plus, once you have established a rapport with a doctor, some PCPs will treat simple problems over the phone at little or even no cost. This presumes you are a regular patient and keep your appointments.

No matter what doctor you choose, you still need to take responsibility, in some ways, for your own health. Most medical studies have found that doctors don't order appropriate tests or prescribe appropriate drugs or even deliver appropriate care about 50 percent of the time!

One of the reasons it is important to ask around for a doctor rather than picking one out of a book is because of who you are and the particular care you might need. For example, you may want your doctor to speak your language of origin. It may also be important for you to have a doctor who understands your particular cultural and ethnic background. Physicians whose practices include large numbers of a particular ethnic group often become very knowledgeable in this regard.

> **Bet You Didn't Know**
>
> A *British Medical Journal* study published in 2007 found that the more time doctors spend talking about themselves during an appointment, the less time the doctor spends listening to the patient. When you leave your appointment, ask yourself: Who was my doctor more interested in? Me or herself?

Another important factor in choosing a primary care physician is to find one whose personal style meshes well with your own. This can be critical when you have to make difficult decisions. You want to find a doctor who is knowledgeable, cares about you as a person, and can communicate well. Doctors are as different as people are in general, so it is worth looking for one who works well with you.

In terms of competence, board certification is at least a baseline measure. You do not need to be board certified to practice medicine, although you do need to graduate from an approved medical school and pass a basic licensing exam.

One way to find the best physicians is to ask a medical professional whom he sees (or would see) for a particular medical issue.

Bet You Didn't Know

Physicians trained in other countries make up about 23 percent of the U.S. physician population. The heaviest concentration of non-US trained physicians is in New Jersey (39.6 percent of doctors); New York (38.6 percent); Florida (33.6 percent); and Illinois (32.3 percent). The largest national group is from India (24.0 percent of total). Some are American citizens who have studied overseas because there are not enough places in U.S. medical schools to accommodate all the students who wish to study medicine.

Finding a Specialist

Besides a primary care doctor, most of us need (or will one day need) one or two *specialists* for specific illnesses. For example, arthritis, diabetes, and mental health issues all require specific treatment and care by specialists. According to the American Board of Medical Specialties, doctors who focus on a particular aspect of patient care are specialists. For example, cardiologists study and see patients with heart problems and heart disease, while endocrinologists focus on the endocrine glands and hormones.

def•i•ni•tion

Specialists are physicians who have received advanced training in a specific area or discipline, such as cardiology (diseases of the heart) or neurosurgery (specialized surgery of the brain and nervous system).

Specialists can concentrate on body systems (nephrologists for the kidneys) or see patients who are in specific age groups, such as pediatricians for children. There are even subspecialists, for example, pediatric nephrologists, who may define their scope of practice even more narrowly. Certain academic research physicians may focus their expertise on new medical and scientific techniques that other physicians need to help diagnose or treat particular medical conditions.

And this is all the more reason you are well advised to have a trusted primary care physician, a family practitioner, internist, or pediatrician, to help you navigate through the world of medical specialists and second opinions.

When you have health insurance, your primary care physician (if you're in a network health program like most people) will recommend which type of specialist you should see. When you don't have health insurance or if you're in a *non-gated* insurance plan, you can decide if and when (and which) specialist you want to see.

> **Bet You Didn't Know**
>
> Most medical specialists study about four to six years longer than general physicians to become eligible for certification in their particular field. This is good news for a patient, but bad news for a wallet as specialists often charge more than primary care doctors.

> **def•i•ni•tion**
>
> A **nongated** insurance plan means you don't need pre-approval from a primary care doctor, in this case known as a "gatekeeper," to have your insurer pay for specialty consultation, so you can decide when and which specialist you see.

Again, bear in mind, you want to make sure you see the right specialist for your symptoms, and that's not always an easy call. Let's say, for example, your symptoms include fatigue, weight gain, and acne. Should you see a specialist? If so, what kind? How do you know if the symptoms are related?

Of course, there are times when you will want to take yourself directly to a specialist. Most likely it will be when you've already been diagnosed with an illness or have long dealt with an ongoing health issue.

Here is a brief description of some of the specialists

◆ An allergist has extensive training in allergy and immunology problems, including asthma, and works with all types of reactions, including skin, sneezing, and other symptoms related to the immune system.

◆ A colo-rectal surgeon diagnoses and treats diseases of the intestinal tract, colon, rectum, and perianal area by surgical means. A gastro-enterologist treats gastrointestinal problems medically and also deals with other organs such as the liver, pancreas, and gallbladder.

◆ A dermatologist diagnoses and treats skin cancers, melanomas, and moles, and manages contact dermatitis and other allergic and nonallergic skin disorders. They also have expertise in the management of cosmetic disorders of the skin, such as hair loss and scars and the skin changes associated with aging.

◆ A pulmonologist focuses on diseases and congenital or structural disorders of the lungs and airways, including cystic fibrosis, chronic obstructive pulmonary disease, recurrent pneumonia, and asthma.

◆ An ophthalmologist has the knowledge and professional skills needed to provide comprehensive eye and vision care. Ophthalmologists are medically trained to diagnose, monitor, and medically or surgically treat all ocular and visual disorders. He may prescribe vision services, including glasses and contact lenses, although often this is done by an optometrist (a non-MD) who also has certain diagnostic and therapeutic training.

◆ An otolaryngologist (OTO) is a head and neck surgeon, although she was once known as an ear, nose, and throat doctor (ENT). These days, OTOs focus on head and neck problems and surgery for the nose, throat, and sinuses.

◆ A neurologist specializes in the diagnosis and treatment of all types of nervous system–related disease or impaired function of the brain, spinal cord, peripheral nerves, muscles, and autonomic nervous system.

◆ A urologist, also known as a genitourinary surgeon, manages congenital and acquired conditions of the genitourinary system (kidneys, ureters, bladder, penis, prostate gland) and contiguous structures including the adrenal gland.

For Your Health _____

If you need to see a specialist, find out if she is board certified, since this means she has studied a specific amount of time in her specialty and has passed an exam about her area of expertise. You can find out if a doctor you see is board certified free of charge. Call 1-866-ASK-ABMS (275-2267), and have the full name of the professional.

Use your instinct when choosing a doctor. And then use your thinking skills after each visit. Do you feel cared for? Do you think your doctor paid attention to your concerns? Did he seem knowledgeable and secure in his diagnosis and treatment?

Even without health insurance, try to coordinate your visit to a specialist through your primary care physician. This will result in better health care and treatment. Likewise, if you think you will need to be hospitalized, try to find both a primary care physician and a specialist who have admitting privileges at your preferred hospital. This gets you access to the specialists and admission at that hospital.

Other issues to consider:

◆ Check to see if your doctor or specialist is up-to-date on any specific problem you have. Simply ask him how he keeps up-to-date on all the new research being done. And if you are talking to a specialist, ask him if he has seen cases like yours before. Ask how much experience he has had in treating patients with your set of symptoms.

◆ Call the state medical board to get more information on your physician. The board can tell you if your doctor has been disciplined or repeatedly sued for malpractice.

◆ Ask your friends and family for recommendations, but also don't hesitate to ask nurses or other professionals within the medical community what they've heard about specific doctors. Ask at your lab or at your pharmacy. Just say "I think I might have [name your specific concern, such as depression or Type 2 Diabetes]. Do you know someone who is good at treating this?"

Do not take Top Doctor or Top Hospital lists in magazines that seriously. Many magazines use criteria that aren't important to an individual patient. Local word of mouth is more reliable than a third-party report unless you can verify what the magazine reports with people whose opinion you can trust.

Organizations and Research

Most major diseases have organizations that do research and help patients who suffer from the illness find doctors. If you suffer from a common or even an uncommon problem, such as arthritis or diabetes, contacting and finding connection with your local chapter of these large national organizations will give you all sorts of valuable information, including physicians who might help you for a lower cost.

Arthritis

Arthritis is a general term that refers to inflammation of the joints. Over 100 different diseases and problems, such as rheumatoid arthritis, juvenile arthritis, and other joint conditions may cause this inflammation that affects around 46 million Americans, according to the Arthritis Foundation.

The Arthritis Foundation is a voluntary organization that works toward finding a cure for these illnesses. It can assist anyone who suffers from arthritis in finding the most up-to-date research, as well as physicians who specialize in their particular type of arthritis. Even more helpful, the organization can guide you to researchers who are looking for people to take part in studies that might provide you with care, as well as the opportunity to further medical knowledge.

Likewise, getting involved in the organization may help you learn more about alternative therapies and treatments that are not only low-cost but also effective. To learn more, go to www.arthritis.org.

Family Risk of Cancer

In 2007, 1.4 million people in the United States were told they had a new case of cancer, and 559,650 people died of the disease. Some cases of cancer are currently unpredictable, but some are known to be genetic (inherited). A small percentage are even known to be caused by a specific single gene. It may be unclear whether a pattern of cancer in a family is caused by a single gene or a combination of genes and risk factors. It is well known, however, that certain specific risk factors significantly increase the chances of contracting cancer. These include: smoking, a diet high in fat, excessive sun exposure, and direct exposure to such carcinogens as benzene (found in gasoline), asbestos, and radiation (found in radon gas in some basements and in cigarette smoke). Cancers sometimes related to a single gene include breast, bowel, colon, melanoma, ovarian, and prostate.

The clues that cancers in the family may be due to an inherited faulty gene include:

◆ The more blood relatives who have developed cancer (in particular, breast, ovarian, and/or bowel cancer), the more likely the cancer is due to an inherited faulty gene.

◆ The younger people are when they develop cancer (compared to what is expected in the general community), the more likely it is to be due to hereditary factors.

◆ The types of cancer and who it affects in the family are important. Particular cancers, such as breast and ovarian cancer or bowel cancer, can run in the family. This happens because some faulty genes can cause more than one type of cancer. (It is important to note that some people who inherit a faulty gene which causes an increased chance of cancer never go on to develop any cancer.)

Abnormalities (mutations) in certain inherited genes have been found to lead to some colon cancers, and two breast cancer genes, BRCA1 and BRCA2, have been discovered in recent years. If you or several relatives have had cancer, were diagnosed under the age of 50, had more than one type of cancer, or had a rare or unusual cancer, then you might be at risk. It might pay for you to have a genetic evaluation to learn more about your health. Go to www.hhs.gov/familyhistory/download.html to learn more about your risk.

Diabetes

Why are more and more people developing diabetes? The simple answer is that a major risk factor for diabetes is caloric overload and resultant obesity, which has become epidemic in America and to a growing degree worldwide. Calories from food are so plentiful, inexpensive, available, and subsidized that even poor people can now easily become obese. As a nation we seem to have won the war on hunger but are, as a result, now fighting the battle of the bulge.

Diabetes results from the inability of the pancreas to provide enough insulin to appropriately handle the metabolism of glucose (sugar). This can result from an insulin deficiency, Type I or "juvenile" diabetes, or from an overwhelming glucose surplus, Type II or "adult"/over-nutrition related diabetes.

Complications of diabetes include heart disease, kidney failure, blindness, dementia, and small blood vessel (vascular) disease which essentially affects every organ system in the body.

Cardiovascular Diseases

Heart disease still kills more people in the United States than any other illness. In fact if you lump together heart disease, stroke, kidney disease, and diabetes (complications of) under the generic label of "vascular diseases" you are looking at close to one million deaths in the United States annually (2004 CDC statistics), with cancer a distant second at 550,000. The good news is that, according to a recent article in *The New England Journal of Medicine*, the death rate from heart disease has dropped an astounding 50 percent over the past twenty years. However, that doesn't mean you're less likely to die because eventual mortality is still 100 percent. It just means you're likely to live longer before you do. Approximately half that reduction is due to prevention and the other half to medical advances and interventions. Perhaps our health care system isn't so bad after all!

The lesson here for everyone, and especially those concerned with health-care costs, is to work hard to control the risk factors for cardiovascular disease. If we as a society would quit smoking, consume fewer calories, keep our blood pressure, cholesterol, and blood sugar (diabetes) under control, we would on average lead longer and healthier lives. We would also save *billions* of dollars on health care in the bargain.

Giving Blood

Decades ago, struggling artists, college students, and medical students would donate blood in order to collect a little money as well as a little bit of food. But people in poor health, such as alcoholics and drug addicts, also donated, and when first hepatitis and then the HIV/AIDS epidemic compromised the blood supply, donation standards tightened significantly.

These days, blood donation does not come with payment as your gift is voluntary. If you truly want to donate for humanitarian reasons, you will get free basic blood tests (a CBC, or complete blood count, and a hepatitis screen) and a glass of juice, but no real health care. You cannot donate if you are less than 110 pounds or have other exclusionary conditions such as a slow heart rate (<50), history of or risk factors for Hepatitis, HIV, malaria, and certain other infectious diseases.

If you are healthy and want to donate blood, though, there are a number of benefits. First and most important, you will be doing a good deed. Second, you will meet some nurses and doctors in the community who may be able to help you find care. Don't be shy about telling people you don't have insurance and are looking for a physician. Simply take the time to say, "I came here today to help, but maybe someone who works here knows what I can do to find health insurance or a doctor who will see me even though I'm not covered." Think of the good you'll be doing in the meantime!

Code Red

Every day, emergency physicians see patients who fake emergencies in order to get treatment for a nonemergency. ER docs say this practice is irresponsible and dangerous because for one thing, it means you may end up having potentially risky and expensive tests and procedures. For another, of course, it may delay care for another person who truly has an emergency, not to mention the added costs to society for unnecessary (and often uncompensated) care.

Clinics

Clinics, which offer free or reduced rates for medical care, are a good resource for someone without insurance. Some patients don't like clinics because they won't see a particular doctor unless they become regular patients. Many teaching hospitals have clinics staffed primarily by residents, doctors in training who are only there for a year or two.

def•i•ni•tion

A **clinic** is an approved public or nonprofit facility organized and operated for the primary purpose of providing outpatient public health services.

On the other hand, clinics often feature a staff filled with physicians who may be highly motivated to provide excellent care, interested in their patients, and not jaded by many years of seeing the same thing over and over. Many community clinics fill a real health care void in their service area. Doctors who work as volunteers in free clinics say the work is often very rewarding despite the lack of monetary payment.

For Your Health

You can dial 2-1-1 in most area codes to get referrals for nonemergency assistance. This connects you to United Way and other local agencies that offer health insurance as well as local health care at reduced prices.

Often your local hospital social service department or emergency department can refer you to a free clinic in your area.

Clinics typically pay doctors less than a private practice, but that doesn't mean the care isn't as good. Some retired physicians work in clinics, and some hospitals support free clinics as a community service. Sometimes the free clinic allows the hospital to decide who needs to be in the emergency department and who simply needs an outpatient visit.

The government subsidizes many local clinics, so go to a government website (www.ask.hrsa.gov/pc) to find a clinic in your area. You pay what you can at these clinics. The wait might be long, but it is possible to develop a relationship with a physician, rather than seeing an emergency physician who may be busy with far more life-threatening situations.

These clinics provide check-ups, care for you when you're sick, care for pregnant women, well-child check-ups and immunizations for children, and, sometimes, dental care and prescription drugs.

At-Home Medical Testing

Blood glucose level tests, pregnancy tests, thyroid tests, more and more people use these at-home medical tests to diagnose or monitor their health conditions. Some are great, easy to use and reliable. But not all of them are trustworthy, and it's important to know if you're getting what you need for your money.

There are three types of at-home tests:

- ◆ Diagnostic: These help to determine if you have a specific health condition, such as pregnancy.

- ◆ Monitoring: These kits monitor health conditions and provide information about whether treatment should be adjusted or if it's working. An example is glucose testing to monitor blood sugar levels in people with diabetes or a sphygmomanometer (blood pressure cuff) to take blood pressure readings.

- ◆ Screens: These let you know if you are in a danger zone for certain diseases, such as testing your blood for cholesterol or triglyceride levels. If you find you have high readings, you might see a doctor to help prevent heart disease.

> **Code Red**
>
> The problem with many tests is that you may get a false-negative or false-positive result. This means, basically, that the result you get is the opposite of the truth. For example, a pregnancy test given too early might read negative when, in fact, you're pregnant. Read the fine print on all at-home tests to understand the likelihood of getting the wrong result.

Certainly these tests, when done right and when reliable, are less expensive and give quicker results than those in labs or with the referral of a physician. However, health and disease are complex. These do-it-yourself tests do not tell you what to do if you find something amiss with your results.

The best and most reliable home tests are endorsed by specific organizations, such as the American Diabetes Association, which prints recommendations on its website about how to choose a good blood glucose monitoring meter (www.diabetes.org/for-parents-and-kids/diabetes-care/BGMeter.jsp).

However, without this helpful information on the proper use of the equipment, it is difficult to know if what you are buying is trustworthy. Certainly, some unsavory companies advertise and sell test kits over the Internet or by mail order. An unlicensed test kit purchased from a foreign supplier very likely is not trustworthy.

Likewise, you cannot rely on results if you don't use the product as instructed. For example, people sometimes try to save money by cutting glucose test strips in half so they will last twice as long, or try to mix and match parts from different kits. Tampering with the contents of a test kit means a reduced likelihood of ending up with accurate results.

There is also a significant chance that people may interpret test results incorrectly. Interpretation of test results should always be part of a comprehensive health assessment.

To minimize errors:

◆ Read the label and directions carefully. Understand exactly what you are supposed to do, and follow the directions to the letter.

◆ Know the limitations of the test.

◆ Remember that, like all medical tests, the results are never 100 percent accurate. Do not take any action or make drastic changes to your treatment based on results without first consulting a physician.

Hospital Hotlines

You're home late at night, and you don't feel well. You can't go to the doctor, but you wish you could run your symptoms by an expert to double-check that you're okay. The answer is to call a hotline.

Many hospitals provide this service free of charge, as it saves them from having patients come in when they don't need to. To find one near you, call your local hospital, and ask if they have a service for residents. These are typically staffed by nurses who will recommend some type of self-care, the name of a physician, or that you come to the hospital immediately.

Bet You Didn't Know

Doctors who subscribe to the service in order to get new patients pay for most of these nurse hotlines. Or hospitals run them as a service to the community. If you or someone in your family is sick, call the hotline and tell them your symptoms. The nurse will then give you advice, such as "Take a fever reducer you can get at the drug store" or "Come to the emergency room" or, even, "You need to see a doctor, and here is a list of some in your area."

You can also go online to sites such as www.healthline.com or www.symptoms.webmd.com to get a sense of what the problem might be. Remember this is not a replacement for care, but you may find that you don't need to visit the emergency department or that, with your new knowledge, you can give the physician you do choose to see more reliable information about your health status.

Used and Trade-ins

Need a wheelchair, crutches, hospital bed, or other piece of medical equipment that would typically be costly or that you might only need for a little while? Try advertising for one on Craigslist, asking a local hospital, or calling nearby charities.

You can go to the Salvation Army to see if they have any on hand, or go to the Resources section of this book (Appendix B) to find various medical supply companies. They all ship equipment around the country, and some specialize in used supplies.

The Least You Need to Know

◆ If you find a doctor you like, be honest with him regarding your insurance status and finances and find out if he's willing to work with you regarding regular payments or getting you health insurance.

◆ Do not diagnose yourself using the Internet, books, or magazines; instead, use this information—if it's reliable—to ask your doctor informed questions.

◆ It is completely possible to get quality health care at a neighborhood drugstore or clinic where the doctors or nurse practitioners should be able to refer you to physicians with more expertise if necessary.

◆ Before you go to the emergency room for a nonemergency problem, call to see if they have a referral line or an outpatient clinic that may help keep you healthy as well as be less expensive in the long run.

◆ You can get medical equipment, such as new or used wheelchairs, online, in local newspapers, or through your doctor's office.

Chapter 6

Women's Health

In This Chapter

- ◆ Women's health is also general health
- ◆ Having a baby?
- ◆ Health programs specific to women
- ◆ Regional women's health offices around the country

Women have certainly come a long way. For generations, aside from midwives, there were no doctors and no medical discipline for women and their health. Researchers and physicians studied men to learn about heart disease, cancer, arthritis, or any other condition, and any findings were thought to apply equally to women. But they don't. Doctors and scientists now know and accept the reality (obvious to some of us long ago) that women's bodies are different from men's. Women have babies; they have a monthly cycle; they react differently than men do to medicines because of hormones and body fat disparities; and they have different emotional needs and ways of connecting with physicians.

Guess what? Health insurance has not kept up with the medical profession. According to a 2007 study by Harvard Medical School, most employers now use high-deductible plans that place an unfair financial burden on women. In general, women need more routine medical tests, and those expenses quickly add up. According to Harvard, "the median expense for men under 45 in these plans was less than $500, but for women it was more than $1,200."

So while women need more health care at a greater cost, they are also less likely to be able to pay for it on their own. This is especially true when women are responsible for the health care needs of children, parents, or other family members—which is a more likely scenario for women than men.

However, because women and their children have higher poverty rates than men, many more of them are covered by Medicaid. But of course, this is only a help for poor women. Middle-income women are far more likely to forego health care altogether since they cannot afford insurance and aren't eligible for public programs. In fact, uninsured women are older, more likely to be married, and more likely to work part-time than men. In addition, women are less likely to have direct access to employer-based health insurance and slightly more likely to purchase individual insurance.

The good news is that there are a number of research facilities, community outreach programs, and organizations designed specifically to help women with all types of health concerns, and not all of them are specifically related to their sex.

Women's Health Programs

If you are a woman and live anywhere near a university or major hospital, you're in luck because many medical schools and hospitals now have specific schools, clinics, or programs dedicated to women's health. And yes, of course, they typically charge their patients or use specific insurance plans, but they are also a great source of health care even for uninsured women.

For example, the University of Michigan Women's Health Resource Center offers, according to its website:

◆ Computer access to reliable consumer health information websites

◆ A lending library with more than 500 books

◆ Pamphlets, handouts, articles, and newsletters on hundreds of health and wellness topics

◆ Educational classes and seminars

◆ Support for breastfeeding mothers

◆ Connection to UMHS programs, services, and physicians

Do you notice the last one? Any woman can go into the resource center and get help connecting with physicians. Does that mean she'll automatically get an appointment? No. Does that mean she won't have to pay for her care? No. But it does mean that the staff is there to help her.

Bet You Didn't Know

Numerous organizations exist for women of specific ethnicities and religions. For example, women can go to the National Asian Women's Health Organization (www.nawho.org), the Latin and Caribbean Women's Health Network (www.reddesalud.org), and the California Black Women's Health Project (www.cabwhp.org). Likewise, there are clinics and clearinghouses for information for Native American and specific Asian populations. To find these services, call the social services department of your local hospital.

Other Health Centers

Michigan, of course, is only one example of a women's health center. Here are three others:

◆ Chicago Women's Health Center, 3435 North Sheffield Avenue, Suite 206A, Chicago, IL 60657; 773-935-6126.

◆ UCSF National Center of Excellence in Women's Health, 2356 Sutter Street, 1st Floor, San Francisco, CA 94143; 415-353-7668.

◆ St Luke's Episcopal Health System, Women's Health Center, 7800 Fannin St., #300, Houston, TX 77054; 713-442-7300.

But there are centers all around the country; in many states you'll find one in each county. Look in your phone book under Women's Health, or call your local hospital to see if it has an affiliated center.

Using the Center

Women's Health Resource Centers have a number of purposes. First, they gather up information for a woman to use when she needs to make health-care decisions. Second, they offer a sympathetic and useful ear for issues specific to women, such as birth control, reproductive health, and breast health. In other words, they'll give you action, not just words.

Classes, of course, are not the same as care from a primary care physician, but if you use the services of these centers regularly and get to know the staff, you will likely benefit from their knowledge and help.

The important thing is to be appreciative of the help these providers give you. In other words, be mindful of both sides of the situation; you are looking for free or low-cost health care and so are a lot of other people who come to the classes and clinics. In other words, these physicians and nurses are busy and fully aware of the insurance problem in this country. Kindness on your part will go a long way in helping you get the care you need and want.

If you can, offer to pay for something, or offer a barter. Maybe the clinic needs a few hours of office help, or maybe they need someone to staff a table at a local wellness day. Become part of the health community, and you may find that health care comes more easily to you.

Sexual Health

In terms of health, what makes women different from men? It's not just their reproductive systems. It's the fact that every other part of their bodies is affected by—or somehow affects—their reproductive system.

Bet You Didn't Know

Having genetic mutations, such as BRCAI or BRCA2, breast cancer genes, cannot be considered pre-existing conditions as a basis for a refusal in health insurance.

In women's bodies, the hormones affect not only the reproductive system, but the cardiovascular system and every other system in ways that it doesn't affect men. And that's because it's not just organs that determine sex, but hormones.

So sexual health is not just about reproduction, but, of course, it does

include birth control. When it comes
to sexual health, women have very
different options depending on what
state they are in.

Because of the women's health movement of the last few years, a number
of free programs and services have
been put into place by the federal,
state, and local governments, as well
as hospitals and clinics, to serve all
women, especially in regard to breast
health and reproductive system
cancers.

> **Bet You Didn't Know**
>
> Some experts believe one
> reason the United States
> could never adopt a single-
> payer health plan is due to
> birth control, abortion, and
> the political arguments that
> surround these issues. Would
> a government-run insurance
> plan cover these medications
> and procedures?

If you are an American Indian, the Indian Social Services Welfare
Assistance will provide financial assistance if you live near or on reser-
vations. Go to www.doi.gov.

If medical expenses are forcing you to choose between housing and
health care, try contacting Projects for Assistance in Transition from
Homelessness (PATH). This organization provides federal grants to
states that partner with local organizations to provide a variety of
health services for homeless people who have serious mental illness.
Contact your local social service agency for more information.

> **Bet You Didn't Know**
>
> Another government-sponsored program for uninsured women is The
> National Breast and Cervical Cancer Early Detection Program (NBC-
> CEDP), which provides free or low-cost mammograms and pap tests for
> women over age 39 who cannot afford breast exams or Pap smears.
> A woman is also covered for cervical cancer screenings if she is at or
> below 250 percent of the federal poverty level and between the ages
> of 18–64. She may also be able to receive clinical breast exams, mam-
> mograms, pap tests, and consultations if the tests are abnormal. Go to
> www.cdc/gov/cancer/nbccedp/contacts.htm, or call 1-888-842-
> 6355. Call early, as there is often a very long wait for appointments.

For Your Health _____

One of the most successful programs, created by the federal govern-ment's Centers for Disease Control, is the Breast and Cervical Cancer Mortality Prevention Act of 1990. This law enables low-income and women at risk to receive tests that will detect breast and cervical can-cer, including breast exams, mammograms, pap tests, and referrals for treatment as well as further testing if a screening outcome is abnormal.

One of the most reliable and trustworthy sources of sexual health care for women is Planned Parenthood. Planned Parenthood began in the early twentieth century and has grown into 111 locally governed groups across the country that operate more than 860 health centers. Each health center provides safe, reliable services including contraception, screening for cancers, and other health testing. Physicians, nurse prac-titioners, and advisors are available to talk with you confidentially.

When it comes to their sexual health, according to Planned Parenthood, women need to be concerned about:

◆ Sexually transmitted diseases

◆ Pregnancy prevention

◆ Unplanned pregnancies

◆ Urinary tract infections

◆ The emotional health of their sexual relationships, i.e., domestic violence or rape.

Planned Parenthood offers help and information for women—and men—on all these topics. Go to www.plannedparenthood.org, and enter your zip code to find a clinic near you.

Pregnancy and Obstetrics Care

Having a baby is an expensive proposition, but skimping on the cost of prenatal care is a mistake. In fact, because it's so important for an expectant mother to take good care of herself and her baby, a number of federal and state programs are designed to help new families with low incomes. And if you are working and don't qualify for those programs, there are other options designed to help you.

First, contact your local hospital as soon as possible (as in, when you find out you are pregnant) and talk to someone in the business office about setting up a payment plan, or ask if they offer a sliding scale of fees associated with *obstetrics*.

def•i•ni•tion

Obstetrics is the medical specialty for pregnancy and delivery.

Many hospitals do offer help to pregnant women because everyone is invested in helping women have healthy babies. If a baby isn't healthy, he will end up in the hospital anyway, at a far higher cost to both consumers and governments.

If you want to get insurance to cover this time of your life, remember, you cannot be refused health insurance because you are pregnant. Pregnancy is not considered a pre-existing condition.

If your pregnancy is uncomplicated, you may wish to look around for a local birthing center. Birth centers provide a complete network of maternity and women's health services, including prenatal care and a laboratory, diagnostic testing and consultation, a midwife's care during labor and birth, and transfer to a hospital if the need arises.

 For Your Health

Birth Center care is covered by major health insurance plans as well as Medicaid in most states, so if you join a state insurance program, inquire about the birth center option.

The estimated cost of a delivery and prenatal care at a birthing center is about $3,000–$4,000, half of what it would be for a delivery at a hospital. Many birth centers also provide sliding scales and payment plans.

To see if you have a local birth center, go to www.birthcenters.org/find-a-birth-center.

Maternal and Child Health Services

State programs provide health care services for low-income women who are pregnant and have children under age 22. The federal government funds these programs and establishes general guidelines regarding services. Each state determines eligibility and identifies the specific services to be provided. For services available in your area, go to performance.hrsa.gov/mchb/mchreports/link/state_links.asp.

Once you have given birth, the best way to feed your baby is through breastfeeding. If you need help, call the National Breastfeeding Helpline, which is staffed by trained breastfeeding counselors who can give you support and encouragement and help you with your basic breastfeeding questions and concerns. Call 1-800-994-9662, or go to womenshealth.gov/breastfeeding.

The LaLeche League also provides breast feeding information and support to new mothers.

Some uninsured or underinsured women make too much money to qualify for government assistance but cannot afford to pay for health insurance or costly medical services, which is a difficult situation for women and their families. However, women in this situation have other options. The following are two such options to consider:

◆ Free clinics. The Free Clinic Foundation of America was founded in 1992 and offers a National Directory of Free Clinics that provide services for the working poor and uninsured. For a list of clinics in your area, call 540-344-8242.

◆ Prescription drug assistance. Some states provide prescription drug assistance to women who are not covered by Medicaid. Also many drug companies will work with your doctor or health-care provider to supply discounted medicines. To learn more, go to www.disabilityresources.org/RX.html.

Women-Specific Health Care

Because women respond to illnesses—as well as treatments and medications—differently than men do, many organizations work specifically to help women.

Women with Cancer

Women who are coping with cancer can find help through a variety of government-sponsored and volunteer organizations. Cancer CARE provides free support, information, financial assistance, and practical help to people with cancer and their families. Low-income and under-served women with breast and cervical cancers can obtain assistance from AVONcares Program for Medically Underserved Women. For more information and a list of more resources, contact the National Cancer Institute at www.nci.nih.gov.

For Your Health

According to the Mayo Clinic, Gardasil is the first vaccine ever designed to prevent a cancer. It specifically works to prevent cervical cancer through stopping the spread of the Human Papilloma Virus (HPV). It only recently became available and is recommended for girls ages 11 to 12, although it may be used in girls as young as age 9. This allows a girl's immune system to be activated before she's likely to encounter HPV through sexual activity.

Women coping with breast cancer can turn to the Susan G. Komen Breast Cancer Foundation at www.komen.org, the world's largest and most progressive grassroots network of breast cancer survivors and activists.

Women with HIV

The federal Ryan White CARE Act funds services for those with HIV/AIDS who are without insurance or financial resources to pay for care. For information about the Ryan White Care Act, call 1-888-275-4772 or go to http://hab.hrsa.gov. Contact your local or state health department to locate a CARE provider in your area.

Women with Autoimmune Diseases

Autoimmune diseases refers to a varied group of more than 80 serious, chronic illnesses that involve almost every human organ system. It includes diseases of the nervous, gastrointestinal, and endocrine systems as well as skin and other connective tissues, eyes, blood, and blood vessels. In all of these diseases, the underlying problem is similar—the body's immune system becomes misdirected, attacking the very organs it was designed to protect.

About 75 percent of autoimmune diseases occur in women, most frequently during the childbearing years. Hormones are thought to play a role because some autoimmune illnesses occur more frequently after menopause, others suddenly improve during pregnancy with flare-ups occurring after delivery, while still others will get worse during pregnancy.

Autoimmune diseases also seem to have a genetic component, but, mysteriously, they can cluster in families as different illnesses. For example, a mother may have lupus erythematosus; her daughter, diabetes; her grandmother, rheumatoid arthritis. Research is shedding light on genetic as well as hormonal and environmental risk factors that contribute to the causes of these diseases.

Autoimmune diseases run the gamut from mild to disabling and potentially life-threatening. To learn more about research and medications specifically about women with autoimmune diseases, to go www.4women.gov/FAQ/autoimmune.htm. Or contact these federal disease-specific centers:

- National Institute of Arthritis and Musculoskeletal and Skin Diseases (NIAMS), NIH, HHS; 1-877-226-4267 or www.nih. gov/about/almanac/organization/NIAMS.htm.

- National Institute of Neurological Disorders and Stroke (NINDS), NIH, HHS; 1-800-352-9424 or www.ninds.nih.gov.

- American Autoimmune Related Diseases Association (AARDA), Inc.; 1-800-598-4668 or www.aarda.org.

- Lupus Foundation of America (LFA), Inc.; 1-800-558-0121 or http://www.lupus.org.

- Thyroid Foundation of America (TFA), Inc.; 1-800-832-8321 or www.tsh.org.

Regional Offices for Women's Health

In 1991 the United States Department of Health and Human Services (HHS) established the Office on Women's Health (OWH), which coordinates the research and information from all the HHS departments involved in women's health. Likewise, the OWH has programs and regional offices designed to help women of all ages and of all incomes.

OWH supports Regional Women's Health Coordinators (RWHCs) in 10 regions. The RWHCs coordinate activities to promote a greater focus on women's health issues at the regional, state, and local levels, including programs in health-care service delivery, research, and the education of the public and health professionals. RWHCs identify regional needs in high-priority health areas, establish networking relationships, and implement initiatives that address regional women's health concerns.

Go to www.4women.gov/owh/about/swhc.cfm to get links to each regional office.

Region I—New England

Region I Women's Health Workgroup (RWHWG) has three Centers of Excellence in Women's Health (COE):

◆ Boston University Medical Center—www.bmc. org/medicine/medicine/Womens_Health

◆ Harvard Medical School—www.health.harvard. edu/Womens_Health

◆ Brown University/Women and Infants Hospital—www. womenandinfants.org/body.cfm?id=624

Region I has two Community Centers of Excellence in Women's Health (CCOE):

◆ Griffin Hospital—www.griffinhealth.org.

◆ Northeastern Vermont Area Health Education Center—www. nevahec.org.

Region I has one Rural/Frontier Women's Health Coordinating Center (RFCC):

◆ North Country Health Consortium, Inc. Go to www.nchin.org to learn more about programs sponsored by this health group.

At these websites, you'll find a lot of health information, but you will also find contact names and numbers to help you get the health care you need.

Each state in the region also has its own program dedicated to women's health.

Connecticut

Connecticut does not have an official Office on Women's Health, and there is no dedicated women's health coordinator position. However, the state has several unique women's health programs, including one which focuses on perinatal depression and related mental health problems in mothers and their families. The "Going Home Healthy" project is a model collaboration between the Connecticut Department of Public Health and the York Correctional Institute (YCI), Connecticut's only women's prison, which brought together government entities and community resources to address transitioning women from the prison back to the community, including access to Social Security and Medicaid prior to release. Connecticut will soon have available an assessment of breastfeeding practices of African American women in the state. For more details on the state's women's health activities go to www.dph.state.ct.

Maine

Maine does not have an official Office on Women's Health; however, it does have a unique government/private sector collaboration on women's health entitled the Maine Women's Health Campaign, which has developed analysis and action plans for comprehensive women's health, adolescent girls' health, and women's cardiovascular health in Maine. It also has a women's health advisory board and an internal women's preventive health group at the Maine Centers for Disease Control. The state has several unique women's health projects, including a program designed to develop successful models for integrated behavioral health in the primary care setting for women of reproductive age; a statewide collaborative group focused on incarcerated women's health; Core Health Indicators for gender-based analysis; the Elder Women's Health Indicators project; and the Caregivers' Survey Project. For more details go to www.maine.gov/dhhs/boh/index.htm.

Massachusetts

Massachusetts does not have an official Office on Women's Health, and there is no dedicated women's health coordinator position. However, the Commonwealth does provide resources for breast cancer screening and research, as well as investigation of environmental factors surrounding breast cancer clusters. The Massachusetts Department of Public health has several unique women's health programs, including The "Stroke Heroes Act FAST" (Face, Arm, Speech, Time) training program, which teaches the subtle symptoms of stroke and fast response; the SANE (Sexual Assault Nurse Examiner) Protocols for persons with disabilities, pediatric cases, and incarcerated persons; the DVSCRIP (Domestic Violence Screening, Care, Referral, and Information Program) training for maternal and child health providers; the Perinatal Connections Project, which aims to increase awareness and decrease stigma associated with perinatal depression and increase access to appropriate mental health services for women and their families; the Batterer's Intervention Program; the "Keep Moving" program for people 50+ ; and the In Situ Breast Cancer and Mammography Licensing Reports. For more details go to www.mass.gov/dph.

New Hampshire

Responsibility for Women's Health Initiatives in New Hampshire is shared between the Manager for Prenatal, Adolescent Health, Abstinence Education, and Injury Prevention Program and the Manager of the State Family Program who also oversees the State's Rape Prevention Education Grant. The state's primary current women's health initiative is a Birth Outcomes Workgroup working toward a coordinated public private-initiative to increase positive birth outcomes by promoting adequate prenatal care and efforts to enhance overall women's health. Other projects have included observation of Women's Health Week over the past three years, the development of a Women's Health Toolkit highlighting basic health promotion messages, and the creation of an Osteoporosis Information Kit. Go to www.nh.gov/csw.

Rhode Island

Rhode Island is the only New England state with an official Office on Women's Health and a full-time, dedicated women's health coordinator. There is also an Office on Women's Health Advisory Committee and an internal workgroup on women's health. The state has several unique women's health programs including an annual women's health conference (The Faces of Women's Health) to increase knowledge of women's health issues among service providers; Health Policy Briefs on various topics, such as Osteoporosis and HIV/AIDS; a Strategic Plan developed by the Advisory Committee with input from Community Forums, and review of an Internal Assessment document. Go to www.health.ri. gov/family/ofyss/fp/index.php.

Vermont

Vermont does not have an official Office on Women's Health nor a dedicated women's health coordinator position. But they do have a Program Director for Breast and Cervical Cancer and *WISEWOMAN* Programs. The state has developed a Women's Health Status Report, a 17-page booklet that includes facts and figures about various trends in women's health care in Vermont. Topics covered include access to care, alcohol and drug use, cancer, diabetes, heart disease, injury and violence, tobacco, obesity, and physical activity. Go to www. healthyvermonters.info.

def•i•ni•tion

> **WISEWOMAN** Programs provide low–income, under– or uninsured 40– to 64–year–old women with the knowledge, skills, and opportunities to improve diet, physical activity, and other lifestyle behaviors to prevent, delay, and control cardiovascular and other chronic diseases. It is administered through CDC's Division for Heart Disease and Stroke Prevention (DHDSP).

Region II

This diverse region has one Women's Health Center of Excellence: The University of Puerto Rico, Medical Science Campus, in San Juan, PR.

New Jersey

The New Jersey Office on Women's Health (OWH) works to raise awareness of women's health issues across the lifespan, serves as a resource for information and referrals, advocates for gender-specific research, develops effective programs to improve women's health, and coordinates with existing programs and organizations that provide health services to the women of New Jersey. Although the Office on Women's Health has only been operational for a few years, the state has a long history of providing health services with a focus on women, including family planning services; prenatal care; breast, cervical, and colorectal cancer screening; and adolescent health services. New Jersey recently unveiled a campaign focused on post-partum depression. Go to www.state.nj.us/health/fhs/owh/index.shtml.

New York

New York State offers a variety of public health programs and services to women. Major components include primary health care, disease prevention and health promotion, early intervention, continuity of care, and elimination of health disparities. As a result of a 2002 grant from the HRSA Maternal and Child Health Bureau, the New York State Department of Health created a profile on statewide women's health programs, with program descriptions and contact information to address heart disease, breast and cervical cancer, diabetes, arthritis, HIV/AIDS, maternal and child health, family planning, rape crisis intervention, and other issues. The New York State Department of Health focuses on health concerns which have direct impact on young, middle age, and older women. Go to www.health.state.ny. us/nysdoh/provider/women.htm.

Region III

The region's demographic, economic, and health status indicators describe a diverse population with challenging needs. The region contains four Centers of Excellence (COE) and one Community Center of Excellence (CCOE) in Women's Health awarded by the Department of Health and Human Services' Office on Women's Health.

Delaware

The state has an Office of Women's Health. Delaware has a National Community Center of Excellence in Women's Health at Christiana Health Care System: www.christianacare.org.

District of Columbia

The District of Columbia has an Office of Women's Health. In the District of Columbia, a Women's Health Initiative is implemented by the Department of Health, Office of Maternal and Child Health. The District's health department's website is www.dchealth.dc.gov. There is no National Centers of Excellence in Women's Health in D.C.

Maryland

Maryland does not have an Office of Women's Health. Go to www. dhmh.state.md.us for available information. There is no National Centers of Excellence in Women's Health in Maryland. Go to www. co.ho.md.us/CitizenServices/ServicesGuide/Women.htm.

Pennsylvania

The state does not have an Office of Women's Health. The state health department website is www.health.state.pa.us/womenshealth. There are two National Centers of Excellence in Women's Health (COE), one at Drexel (www.drexelmed.edu/iwhl/COPE.asp) and the other at Magee (www.magee.edu/coe/homepage/home.html).

Virginia

There is no Office of Women's Health in the Virginia Department of Health. The state health department website is www.vdh.state.va.us. Virginia also has a nonprofit organization Women's Health Virginia which provides educational programs on women's health. The website for this organization is www.womenshealthvirginia.org. Virginia has a National Centers of Excellence in Women's Health at Virginia Commonwealth University, www.womenshealth.vcu.edu.

West Virginia

There is no Office of Women's Health, but the state health department's website is www.wvdhhr.org/bph. West Virginia has a Center

of Excellence in Women's Health at West Virginia University, www.
wvhealthywomen.org.

Region IV

Region IV includes Alabama, Florida, Georgia, Kentucky, Mississippi,
North Carolina, South Carolina, and Tennessee. One Center of Excel-
lence (COE) in Women's Health is at the University of Mississippi in
Jackson, Mississippi and another Women's Health Center of Excellence
is at the Wake Forest University Baptist Medical Center, Winston-
Salem, North Carolina. There are three Community Centers of
Excellence (CCOE) in Birmingham, Alabama; Clearwater, Florida; and
Atlanta, Georgia. There are two Rural Frontier Coordinating Centers
(RFCC) in Madisonville, Tennessee; and Jackson, Kentucky.

By the year 2010, more than 10 percent of the population will live in
Region IV, and Florida will be the third largest state in the nation.
The key health issues facing Region IV are not unlike those issues that
other regions and the nation are facing. The key health issues are access
to quality health services, breast and cervical cancer, domestic violence,
high teen pregnancy rates, high infant mortality, mental health and
substance abuse, and chronic disease, such as heart disease, stroke, and
diabetes.

Alabama

Alabama does have an official Office on Women's Health with
a dedicated women's health coordinator position. Go to www.
womenshealthlink.net for the Cooper Green Hospital as a National
Community Center of Excellence in Women's Health.

Florida

Florida has an official Office on Women's Health and a dedicated
women's health coordinator position (with no contact information or
website). There is a Community Center of Excellence in Clearwater,
www.turleyccoe.org.

Georgia

Georgia has an official Office on Women's Health and a women's
health coordinator's position. Georgia's Office of Women's Health

services is one of four population teams located in the Family Health Branch of Georgia's Division of Public Health. Within the Office of Women's Health Services are the state's family planning, perinatal health, and women's health programs. The major goal of the Office of Women's Health Services is to establish a comprehensive community-based system of care. Go to http://health.state.ga.us/programs/women and a Community of Excellence, www.oakhurstmedical.org.

Kentucky

Kentucky has an official Office on Women's Health. Women's Health Programs are Abstinence Education, Adolescent Health/Positive Youth Development, Breast and Cervical Cancer Screenings, Family Planning/Reproductive Health, Folic Acid Supplementation, and Pre-conception Care. Go to http://chfs.ky.gov/dph/info/wpmh.

Mississippi

The Mississippi Department of Health's Office of Women's Health provides and ensures access to comprehensive health services that affect positive outcomes for women, including early cancer detection, domestic violence, osteoporosis screening, prevention and intervention, family planning, and maternity services. Maternity services include perinatal risk management for infants (PHRM), a Medicaid program designed to decrease infant mortality and low birth weight infants by providing quality health care to pregnant women. Efforts are often collaborated with the Center of Excellence for Women at the University of Mississippi Medical Center. For more information, go to www.msdh.state.ms.us/msdhsite/_static/41.html.

North Carolina

Because of a lack of funding, the Office of Women's Health no longer functions. Since 1997, the Women's Health Branch within the Division of Public Health handles inquiries. Go to wch.dhhs.state.nc.us/whs.htm. Local health departments in each of the 100 counties provide a variety of services to improve women's health, such as family planning, prenatal care, flu shots and other women's immunizations, and maternity care coordination.

South Carolina

For details on women's health activities go to www.scdhec.net, then click on "Health," then "Maternal, Child Health." The web URL is incredibly long, but using those clicks will take you to an excellent directory. Or call 1-800-868-0404.

Tennessee

Tennessee has an official Office on Women's Health, and the women's health coordinator position also serves as the director of the Women's Health/Genetics Section of the Tennessee Department of Health. There is also a women's health advisory committee. The Department has many programs that provide services for women. Go to www. health.state.tn.us/womenshealth/index.htm to learn more.

Region V

This region, the largest of the ten, represents almost 18 percent of the total U.S. population with over 50 million inhabitants. Health issues of concern to women in Region V are similar to those of women all across the country and include, but are not limited to, access to care, poverty, domestic and all forms of violence, cardiovascular disease, smoking, physical inactivity, substance abuse, poor nutrition, mental health, disparities among various racial and ethnic groups, sexually transmitted diseases including HIV and AIDS, and a shortage of health-care providers adequately trained to provide care that is both appropriate and sensitive to the needs of women. Five of the twenty designated National Centers of Excellence in Women's Health (COE) are located in the region. Go to www.4woman.gov/coe/centers to learn more about all of them.

Illinois

Illinois has a state-funded Office of Women's Health, and a designated Center of Excellence on Women's Health is at the University of Illinois at Chicago; go to www.uic.edu/orgs/womenshealth. There is also a solid foundation of poorly funded, yet very effective nonprofit organizations that provide direct services, such as the Chicago Women's Health Center, which has an established women-centered practice and other grassroots efforts, such as the Women's Health Education Project and the Illinois Women's Health Coalition, which works to impact health policy related to women. Go to www.ilmaternal.org/AboutUs.htm.

Indiana

Indiana has a designated National Centers of Excellence in Women's Health (CoE) at Indiana University School of Medicine, Indianapolis (www.iupui.edu/~womenhlt) and a state-funded Office on Women's Health (www.in.gov/isdh/programs/owh).

Michigan

The Michigan Department of Community Health (MDCH), www.michigan.gov/mdch, has a wide variety of women's health programs promoting women's health issues which focus on access to care and prevention. Following is a list of women's health programs within MDCH: Family Planning, Substance Abuse Demonstration Projects, Fetal Alcohol Syndrome Maternal and Child HIV/AIDS Program, Maternal and Infant Health Advocacy Services Program, Maternal Support Services, Prenatal Care Outreach and Advocacy Program, Prenatal Care Clinic Program, Prenatal Smoking Cessation, Women, Infants, and Children Program, Breastfeeding Peer Counselor Initiative, Farmer's Market, Priorities of the Michigan Cancer Consortium, Violence Against Women Prevention Program, Women's Cancer Screening Program in Michigan, Michigan Steps Up Healthy Lifestyle Campaign, and Women's Designated Services Program. The University of Michigan Health System, Ann Arbor is a designated National Centers of Excellence in Women's Health; go to www.med.umich.edu/whp.

Minnesota

Minnesota has a designated Center of Excellence in Women's Health at the University of Minnesota, Minneapolis and a Community Center of Excellence in Women's Health at Hennepin Primary Care Department, Minneapolis. Go to www.womenshealth.wisc.edu.

Ohio

NorthEast Ohio Neighborhood Health Services, Inc. in Cleveland is a designated Community Center of Excellence (CCoE) in Women's Health; go to www.nhlink.net/ClevelandNeighborhoods/hough/neon/NEON.htm or www.odh.ohio.gov/odhPrograms/odhPrograms.aspx.

Wisconsin

The Women's Health Officer works closely with the nonprofit Wisconsin Women's Health Foundation, a designated Rural Frontier Coordinating Center, on a variety of health education projects, including a smoking cessation program for pregnant women. Wisconsin is also home to one of the National Centers of Excellence in Women's Health at the University of Wisconsin, Madison. Go to www.wwhf.org or www.womenshealth.wisc.edu.

Region VI

This region has five states: Arkansas, Louisiana, New Mexico, Oklahoma, and Texas. The key health issues affecting the region are heart disease, lack of prenatal care, breast and cervical cancer, diabetes, HIV/AIDS, intimate partner violence, and lack of health insurance.

Arkansas

Go to www.healthyarkansas.org to learn more about programs.

Louisiana

Go to www.4women.gov/owh/reg/6/louisiana.cfm. There is a National Centers of Excellence in Women's Health at Tulane/Xavier Universities, www.tulane.edu/~tuxcoe/NewWebsite.

New Mexico

Go to www.health.state.nm.us/OPMH/OPMHW.htm or www.4women.gov/owh/reg/6/newmexico.cfm to learn more about programs.

Oklahoma

The state women's health liaison works with many diverse groups and recently partnered with the National Indian Women's Health Resource Center in Tahlequah to host a Tribal Young Women's Health Summit for tribes in Oklahoma and Louisiana. She works with the Oklahoma American Heart Association concerning women's heart health and the University of Oklahoma Medical Center on areas of gynecological health, especially breast and cervical cancer. She is concerned about older women's health, especially osteoporosis and incontinence problems. She works to address women's health inequities and supports community activities in the area of women's health promotion/prevention activities. Go to www.health.state.ok.us/program/mchs.

Texas

The women's health team is working to improve women's health and will be focusing on professional physician training throughout the state concerning Perinatal HIV/AIDS Management. They will partner with the state ACOG chapter and will be using the national ACOG training materials. Go towww.forwoman.gov/owh/reg/6/texas.cfm

Region VII

Region VII includes Iowa, Kansas, Missouri, and Nebraska. The female population is mostly white with all the states having 10 percent or less of their female population comprised of women of color. Some key women's health issues are access to care, cardiovascular disease, domestic violence, HIV/AIDS, mental health services, substance abuse services, breast cancer, health education needs, and language and culture as barriers to services. There is a Center of Excellence in Women's Health at the University of Missouri—Kansas City Medical School, in Kansas City, Missouri and two Community Centers of Excellence at Greeley Health Services in Tribune, Kansas and Northeast Missouri Health Council, Inc. in Kirksville, Missouri.

Iowa

The Iowa Department of Public Health (IDPH) has an Office on Women's Health. Go to www.idph.state.ia.us/resources.asp and www.womenshealthiowa.info.

Kansas

The Kansas Department of Health and Environment (KDHE) does not have an official Office on Women's Health; however, they do have a women's health coordinator. The state sponsors several women's health programs including the Early Detection Works program, which screens for Breast and Cervical Cancer. This program emphasizes the importance of breast self exams, mammograms, and clinical breast exams. The Disability program focuses on preventing secondary conditions and promoting the health of people with disabilities. Five priorities have been identified. One of the five is violence and abuse of people with disabilities, primarily women. For more details go to www. KDHEKS.gov and www.preventionworkskansas.com.

Missouri

The Missouri Department of Health and Senior Services (DHSS) has an official Office on Women's Health and a full-time dedicated women's health coordinator. The state has several women's health projects within the Show me Healthy Women program, including the WISE-WOMEN and Breast and Cervical Control Project. These programs address breast and cervical as well as cardiovascular disease and prevention, particularly among low-income women. Missouri developed a state strategic plan to prevent violence against women.

Nebraska

The Nebraska Department of Health and Human Services (DHHS) has an official Office on Women's Health and a full-time dedicated women's health coordinator. The state has several women's health programs including Every Woman Matters and the WISEWOMAN program. Every Women Matters focuses on breast and cervical cancer and the importance of early detection through screening. WISE-WOMAN focuses on cardiovascular disease and the importance of early detection of heart disease and breast cervical cancer, particularly among low-income women. The Colorectal Screening Program will be integrated into Everywoman Matters. It focuses on prevention and early detection of colon cancer. Go to www.hhss.ne.gov/hew/OWH.

Region VIII

This region includes Colorado, Montana, North Dakota, South Dakota, Utah, and Wyoming. Women in Region VIII are primarily white. American Indian women and Latinas are the largest minority populations. In addition, this region is very much a rural and frontier area with only a few large metropolitan areas. Some key women's health issues here are heart disease, stroke, cancers, access to care, mental health, suicide, domestic violence, and substance abuse.

Colorado

Colorado does not have an official Office on Women's Health. There is a Rural and Frontier Coordinating Center at the Colorado Coalition for the Homeless. One unique program is a social marketing campaign to promote adequate weight gain during pregnancy called *A Healthy Baby is Worth the Weight*. Consumers and providers are both targeted. Go to www.cdphe.state.co.us/cdphehom.asp.

Montana

Montana does not have an Office on Women's Health. The current coordinator is the Health Education Specialist in the Men's and Women's Health Section, which primarily focuses on the *Title X* grant program. Many small contracts have been awarded in Montana related to women's health, including health fairs for National Women's Health Week, educational programs on osteoporosis, heart disease, and eating disorders. There is a Pick Your Path to Health project with the Morning Stars Circle of Women.

def•i•ni•tion

> For more than 30 years, **Title X** has been the nation's major program to reduce unintended pregnancy by providing contraceptive and related reproductive health care services to low-income women. Although public funds for family planning services also come from other programs— including Medicaid, state funds, Temporary Assistance for Needy Families (TANF), State Children's Health Insurance Program (SCHIP), and the Maternal and Child Health and Social Services block grants—Title X is the only federal program dedicated solely to funding family planning and related reproductive health care services.

For more details on this state's women's health activities, go to www. dphhs.mt.gov.

North Dakota

North Dakota does not have an Office on Women's Health. Statewide programs focused on women's health include statewide listings of services for women and children and a newsletter for new mothers. There is a National Centers of Excellence in Women's Health demonstration project at the University of North Dakota. Go to www.und.nodak.edu/dept/womeshealth or www.health.state.nd.us.

South Dakota

South Dakota does not have an Office on Women's Health. The current coordinator is the coordinator for the All Women Count program, a WISEWOMAN project. There is a National Centers of Excellence in Women's Health demonstration project at the University of South Dakota. Go to www.usd.edu/med/ruralhealth/coe.cfm or go to www.state.sd.us.doh.

Utah

Utah has no Office on Women's Health. The current coordinator is the manager of the reproductive health program and part of the *Title V* block grant program. Several women's health projects in Utah include Go Red for Women project and several small contracts for National Women's Health Week. There is a National Centers of Excellence in Women's Health demonstration project at the University of Utah and a Rural/Frontier Coordinating Center at Utah Navaho Health Services. Go to http://health.utah.gov.

> **Bet You Didn't Know**
>
> **Title V** was part of the Social Security Act, made federal law in 1935, which created the Maternal and Child Health Service programs. Block grants allocate monies specifically for programs that improve the health of mothers and children.

Wyoming

Wyoming does not have an Office on Women's Health. The current coordinator is manager of the perinatal systems program, located in the Maternal and Child Health/Title V program. The state is working on a five-year needs assessment project that includes women's health. There is a Rural/Frontier Coordinating Center at the Wyoming Health Council. Go to www.wdh.state.wy.us/main/index.asp.

Region IX

Region IX is the most populous as well as racially, ethnically, and culturally diverse region in the United States. Of the total regional population of 40,174,513 over 40 percent are people of color, which is more than twice the national average. And in major urban cities, such as San Francisco, it is not unusual for more than 100 different languages to be spoken.

The region is home to three National Centers of Excellence in Women's Health:

◆ University of California at San Francisco

◆ University of California at Los Angeles

◆ University of Arizona Health Sciences Center at Tucson.

There are two National Community Centers of Excellence in Women's Health:

◆ Mariposa Community Health Center in Nogales, Arizona

◆ Kokua Kalihi Valley Comprehensive Family Services in Honolulu, Hawaii.

There are also two Rural/Frontier Coordination Centers for Women's Health:

◆ Arizona Association of Community Health Centers in Phoenix

◆ Southern Nevada Area Health Education Center in Las Vegas.

Arizona

"Migrant streams," the agricultural routes which Mexican migrant workers follow to earn a living, result in key state health issues. The results are difficulties in follow-up care, lack of preventive health care, and similar issues, especially for women. The Office of Women's and Children's Health, within the Arizona Department of Health Services, has primary responsibility for the health of women and children in the state.

California

The major health concerns are HIV/AIDS, teen pregnancy, breast cancer, cardiovascular disease, and infant mortality. The Office of Women's Health serves as the focal point within the department for setting and monitoring women's public health policies, promoting more comprehensive and effective approaches to improve women's health, including better coordination of existing programs and resources, and enhancing the visibility and prominence of women's health problems as well as innovative solutions.

Hawaii

Hawaii is the only state in the U.S. which devotes an entire month to promoting women's health prevention and education. The Hawaii State Commission on the Status of Women in collaboration with the Department of Health and other agencies and organizations throughout the state launches a "Women's Health Month" each September. The Governor signs an annual proclamation, and each island holds health fairs, lectures, and special activities which address the health concerns of women and promote healthy lifestyles. Over 400 activities which focus on women's health are held throughout the state. The Family Health Services Division is the departmental unit which has the lead responsibility for women's health issues. One of these is the maternal mortality death rate, which is higher than the rest of the United States. Other departmental focuses are on reducing the pregnancy rate in late teens, 17–19 years old and promoting violence prevention activities.

Nevada

The Bureau of Family Health Services is the focal point within the Nevada State Health Division for women's health issues. The Bureau has 110 employees and 12 different programs. It administers all of the Title V programs, such as WIC and Newborn Screening. With the second highest teen pregnancy rate in the United States, a major focus of women's health activities has rested with Title V initiatives and pregnancy. The Bureau is involved in prevention activities, i.e., media campaigns such as "Baby Your Baby?", teen leader programs, and the Youth Advisory Council. The result has been a recent 6.3 percent decrease in the teen pregnancy rate. Moreover, the Health Division has received a Breast and Cervical Cancer Early Detection Program grant. The state holds a "First Lady's Conference on Women's Health Issues," a collaborative biennial effort between the Southern Nevada AHEC, the State Health Division, and the Governors' Spouse.

Region X

Region X comprises Alaska, Idaho, Oregon, and Washington. This is the largest region in area, but with the smallest population.

Alaska

Alaska is the largest state in the United States with over 586,412 square miles of land area. The total population is estimated at 626,932, by the 2000 census, for a population density of only 1.06 persons per square mile. Many communities, particularly in the Southeast part of the state, are accessible only by air or water routes known as Alaska's Marine Highway. Most pubic health services are provided by federally subsidized native health corporations (for eligible beneficiaries), private nonprofit agencies, or directly by state-employed staff. There are two independent health departments in Alaska.

The Alaska Division of Public Health (DPH) supports a Women's Health Unit in the Section of Women's, Children's, and Family Health. Go to www.hss.state.ak.us/dph/wcfh. Priority activities in 2005–2006 include the creation of an abortion/pregnancy/contraception information website, maintaining the Title X Family Planning Program in geographic areas with proven high incidence of unintended pregnancy, and improving coordination of women's health activities occurring throughout the department and/or division to reduce duplication of efforts.

Idaho

The primary providers of public health services are the seven public health districts. They cover multiple counties and are governed by local boards appointed by the county commissioners within each district. Women's health issues include access to care for rural women, domestic violence, increasing awareness of preventive care needs of women, especially for older women, and access to appropriate prenatal care. The Idaho State Department of Health and Welfare, Division of Health has a variety of public health programs addressing the needs of Idaho women. These efforts include family planning, sexually transmitted diseases and HIV, breast and cervical health, diabetes, physical activity and nutrition, maternal and child health (MCH), Women, Infant, and Children Nutrition Program, injury prevention, and general health promotion.

Oregon

In Oregon, 19 percent of women smoke, 33 percent have been diagnosed with high cholesterol, 20 percent report that they engage in no physical activity, 21 percent report they are obese, 15 percent report they have no health-care coverage, and more than 20 percent of eligible Oregon women don't get routine mammograms. Medical insurance in Oregon has been available to all resident families with incomes to 100 percent of Federal Poverty Level (FPL). Pregnant women with incomes to 185 percent FPL are eligible for Medicaid benefits through the Oregon Health Plan (OHP). In addition, through the Family Planning Expansion Project, all Oregonians of reproductive age with incomes to 185 percent FPL have access to comprehensive family planning services.

Washington

In looking at chronic diseases that affect women, Washington has the highest rate of occurrence of breast cancer in the country, although death rates are slightly below the national average. There is also a "stroke buckle or belt" in the Pacific Northwest for stroke. The state has the eighth highest stroke rate in the country with more women dying from stroke than men in absolute numbers, although this is not reflected in death rates. Heart disease remains the leading cause of death. Asthma is another chronic condition that affects women disproportionately starting in their teen years and throughout adulthood.

For more information on the Washington women's health program, visit www.doh.wa.gov/cfh/WHRN.

Programs for Women With Children (WIC)

Women, Infants, and Children, or WIC, is a federal agency that oversees the health of low-income women, infants, and children under the age of five. WIC can provide you and your family with help to purchase nutritious foods. Their program will not allow you to buy junk food or foods that are unhealthy. Plus, WIC will help you get information on how to eat well and can provide you with referrals to health care. Go to www.fns.usda.gov/wic.

Also look in Chapter 7 as many programs serve both children and their mothers. In other words, getting care for your children may also give you a way to get care for yourself.

Keep Yourself Healthy

Women are notorious for not taking care of themselves because they are busy taking care of others, especially the people they love. But experts have long said that the best thing women can do for those they love is take care of themselves. Healthy, happy women make the healthiest, happiest moms, daughters, sisters, and friends.

The Least You Need to Know

- ◆ Many programs, geared specifically to women, include community clinics and national programs, so call state health departments to find out about specific women's issues.

- ◆ Women's health issues are often thought to be only related to the reproductive system, but the leading causes of death for women are heart disease and non-breast cancers, including lung, so all women need to be aware of the risk factors for those diseases.

- ◆ Young women in particular need to be encouraged to begin to adopt healthy lifestyles, including not smoking, wearing seatbelts, using pregnancy and STD protection, having regular checkups, and exercising and eating well.

- ◆ Keeping yourself healthy and happy, if you're a woman and a mom, should be as much a priority as keeping your family healthy and happy.

Chapter 7

Children's Health

In This Chapter

- ◆ Welcome to the world!
- ◆ Finding a pediatrician
- ◆ Wellness and immunizations
- ◆ Public Health Programs

According to 2005 United States census statistics, 8.3 million children (people under the age of 18) do not have health insurance. This number represents about 12 percent of the entire child population.

Children without health insurance are less likely to:

- ◆ Receive needed shots that prevent disease.
- ◆ Get treatment for recurring illnesses, such as ear infections and asthma.
- ◆ Get preventative care to keep them well.
- ◆ Get the treatment they need when they are sick.

Uninsured children do not just suffer during their younger years; the effects of inferior health care follow them as they get older. Children who aren't treated for chronic illness such as asthma develop poor eating habits, lack exercise, miss correct immunizations, and don't receive proper dental care are at risk to grow up to be adults who are in poor health.

Although free clinics and wellness opportunities are available for children to get health care without having health insurance, most states try to insure children because it is the best way to help them stay healthy and get the care they need.

One of the most disturbing aspects of the problem of children without health insurance is that, according to the AAP, almost 75 percent of uninsured children are actually eligible for government-issued insurance, such as SCHIP, Medicaid, or Title XXI programs, all of which we'll explain in this chapter. Of course, it is disturbing that about 30 percent of uninsured children aren't eligible for any government program, but if the other 75 percent were covered, the nation's children would benefit greatly.

Healthcare for Newborns

Alarmingly, American children have the second highest infant mortality rate in the modern world, according to the United Nations. American babies are three times more likely to die in their first month as children born in Japan, and infant mortality is 2.5 times higher in the United States than in Finland, Iceland, or Norway.

Hopefully you found a way to get appropriate health care during your pregnancy (see Chapter 6), but, if you didn't and now find yourself with a newborn, we encourage you to look into federal and state-funded programs for your baby.

If you do have health insurance, newborns and adopted children may not be excluded for preexisting conditions if they are enrolled in a health plan within 30 days of birth or adoption. Also under the Newborns' and Mothers' Health Protection Act, if a plan covers maternity or newborn benefits, it must allow mothers and newborns a 48-hour hospital stay after a vaginal birth and 96 hours for a cesarean section unless the physician and mother agree on an earlier discharge.

If you deliver in the hospital, the 48-hour period or 96-hour period starts at the time of delivery. So for example, if a woman goes into labor and is admitted to the hospital at 10 P.M. on June 11 but gives birth by vaginal delivery at 6 A.M. on June 12, the 48-hour period begins at 6 A.M. on June 12.

However, if you deliver outside the hospital and are later admitted to the hospital in connection with childbirth as decided by the attending provider, the period begins at the time of the admission. So, for example, if a woman gives birth at home by vaginal delivery but begins bleeding excessively in connection with childbirth and is admitted to the hospital, the 48-hour period starts at the time of admission.

One of the biggest problems with births and newborns in terms of a lack of insurance is the length of a hospital stay. When the Institute of Medicine studied hospital discharge data, it found that a lack of health insurance was associated with "an elevated and increasing risk of adverse outcomes in newborns." In fact, the institute states, "We believe that the elevated and increasing risks for uninsured newborns are explained at least in part by inadequate and diminishing access to care and that this burden is borne disproportionately by blacks and Latinos."

No matter what your insurance status, if you go to the hospital to have a baby, the hospital will deliver the baby, although you may not get the care an insured person would receive. Likewise, you can't be sure your child will get the screening tests a newborn should have.

According to the March of Dimes, all states screen newborns for phenylketonuria (PKU) and congenital adrenal hyperplasia (CAH). All states except three (Louisiana, Pennsylvania, and Washington) screen for galactosemia. Most screen for Sickle Cell Disease. Other screens that vary from state to state are Maple Syrup Urine Disease (21 states),

Homocystinuria (14 states), Biotinidase Deficiency (22 states), Toxoplasmosis (New Hampshire and Massachusetts), Cystic Fibrosis (6 states), Tyrosinemia (Georgia), HIV (New York), MCAD (Massachusetts, Maine, North Carolina, Wisconsin), G6PD (Washington, D.C.), and/or universal hearing screening (27 states).

According to the Save Babies Through Screening Foundation, all newborns receive comprehensive Newborn Screening (NBS) for 50+ disorders in Minnesota, Mississippi, and Washington, D.C., and have the option in Nebraska. Almost all babies receive screening in Pennsylvania. Likewise, various hospitals across the United States. contract with a private laboratory for supplemental NBS totaling 50+ disorders.

> **Bet You Didn't Know**
>
> The average cost of having a baby is $6,378 for a normal delivery and $10,638 for a cesarean.

Save Babies Through Screening (www.savebabies.org) has a limited number of newborn screening packets available each month, free of charge, for expectant parents who qualify. Parents who reside in most states of the United States and who are not able to pay for a supplemental newborn screening packet are eligible.

To get a packet, you must apply early in your third trimester (seventh month of your pregnancy) to arrange with your hospital for a few extra drops of blood to be drawn from your baby's heel at the same time as the routine newborn screening specimen is taken. It is not advisable to simply show up for delivery and unexpectedly hand over the packet. Hospital personnel are not necessarily familiar with supplemental newborn screening and may refuse. At the very least, they may need time to put the procedure in place, so it's best to alert them several weeks before your baby's due date.

Call 1-888-454-3383, mention "free newborn screening packet," and leave your name and phone number.

After the newborn screening, your baby should first see his pediatrician when he is two weeks old. The doctor will check the baby's weight, height, and head circumference. He will probably have a repeat of his newborn screen test and may get his first vaccine.

Well Child Visits

A school-age child ideally should have physical exams every year done by a pediatrician who knows him and has watched him develop. Well-child visits give your child's doctor a chance to track development and ensure that he is getting immunizations on time. In short, it is in your child's best interest to find a pediatrician who will see him on a regular basis.

A pediatrician will look for congenital conditions, spinal alignment, vision problems, subnormal or abnormal growth and development patterns, as well as signs for any chronic conditions, such as allergies, asthma, or diabetes.

Code Red

Do not bring your baby to the emergency room for a well-child visit or a check-up. While it may seem obvious, you need to know, there are sick people in a hospital, and your child is vulnerable to diseases. Instead, call the hospital to see if they have a free clinic or physician who will make sure your baby is healthy.

Supporting your child's relationship with his pediatrician will help him as he gets older, as teenagers often turn to trusted adults outside the family when dealing with problems such as depression, anxiety, substance abuse, and peer pressure.

To find a pediatrician, call your local hospital or look in the phone book. Ask for referrals at pharmacies or at your child's daycare or school. You can also go to the website of the American Academy of Pediatrics, www.aap.org. This website will give you reliable health information, including vaccination schedules. Also look for a red link saying "Find a Pediatrician," and click on that to find a doctor.

For Your Health

Bringing your child to the doctor is a way to model good self-care, i.e., good health habits that your child will take with him as he becomes an adult. Taking the time to go to the doctor will prove to your child that he is worth the time and money good health requires.

Vaccinations

It is very important that children receive vaccinations to protect them against many childhood diseases. And the state requirements for vaccinations continue to change annually. For example, in late 2007, New Jersey began to require that preschoolers get a flu vaccine each year.

A study published in the *Journal of the American Medical Association* and conducted at Harvard Medical School found that for children whose health insurance doesn't cover newly recommended shots, it may be better to pay for them yourself in cash. You may also wish to appeal this decision to your insurance carrier and consider changing to a different policy. Free vaccines are available to children who are uninsured or qualify for public insurance. But the study found that many states can't afford to help children with inadequate private insurance that doesn't cover new, expensive shots and even some older shots, which puts more than a million children at risk. About 55 million employees and their dependents get coverage through self-insured companies that are exempt from state mandates. Those people are the most likely to be underinsured for vaccines.

Illinois, for example, doesn't provide vaccines against chickenpox, pneumonia, hepatitis A, and human papilloma virus to children with insufficient private insurance, so parents would have to pay $400 out of pocket for those vaccines. Vaccinations are among the most cost-effective strategies known to modern medicine and are one of the major reasons that average life expectancy in the United States increased from around 40 at the turn of the century to age 78 by 2004. Even if you have to forgo some of life's little luxuries like that morning cup of coffee and especially cigarettes, alcohol, and breakfast at the fast-food joint, vaccinations are worth paying for. After all, they are for the health of your children. Remember, you always have the option to pay out of pocket

> **Bet You Didn't Know**
>
> Childhood shots have become a billion-a-year dollar endeavor for government since the discovery of polio vaccine 55 years ago. The per-child cost grew more than sevenfold from $155 in 1995 to $900 for boys and $1,200 for girls this year. Costs in the private sector are higher.

for vaccinations and tests your doctor recommends. Often you can be reimbursed by the insurance company if you appeal an initial denial.

Sixteen states require health insurers to cover all recommended vaccines. Workers covered by plans marketed by Aetna and other insurance companies generally are covered for childhood vaccines although they may have to pay co-payments or satisfy deductibles.

Recommended standard vaccines protect children against Diphtheria, Haemophilus influenza type B, Hepatitis B, Measles, Mumps, Rubella, Pertussis, Poliomyelitis, Tetanus, Varicella, and Pneumococcal disease. According to the Centers for Disease Control and Prevention's (CDC) National Immunization Program, approximately one in four children in the United States newborn to 2-year-olds are not properly immunized against infectious diseases.

Children through the age of 18 are eligible if they fall into one of the following categories:

- ◆ Enrolled in Medicaid

- ◆ Uninsured

- ◆ Underinsured (insurance does not cover immunizations)

- ◆ American Indian/Alaskan Native

- ◆ Enrolled in CHIP

For Your Health

No vaccine is more important than another. In fact, the U.S. Centers for Disease Control and Prevention oppose prioritizing vaccines. They have instead called for insurers and the government to provide equal accessibility for recommended vaccines.

You can download an immunization schedule from numerous government websites, including www.aap.org/healthtopics/immunizations.cfm and www.cdc.gov/vaccines/recs/schedules/downloads/child/2007.

Public Health Programs

Public health insurance provided to children is free or low-cost. The costs are different depending on the state and a family's income, but when there are charges, they are minimal. In some states, parents may need to pay a premium or co-payment for their children's health insurance. Most states cover children up to their nineteenth birthday with family incomes of up to $34,100 a year for a family of four. Some states cover children whose families have higher incomes. Income and family size will determine whether or not children qualify.

Most states have made it very easy for parents to apply for health insurance for their children; often the application is very short and can be completed through the mail or over the phone without having to take time off work. Call 1-877-KIDS NOW if you have any questions about filling out the application.

> **Bet You Didn't Know**
>
> Many state health insurance programs for children provide them with vision and dental care, too. Likewise, many schools will offer free screenings to children. These screenings will put you in touch with eye doctors and dentists who will help children without insurance.

Parents and other household members cannot be required to give their social security numbers to get health insurance for their children, but they may be asked to provide social security numbers for their children who are applying for coverage.

Nor do parents and other household members have to give any information about their immigration status to get health insurance for their children. They may be asked to list the people in the household because this information is used to determine the size of the family. Only immigration status information for those children who are applying for coverage must be provided.

Parents will have to give information about the family's income. In some states, they also may be asked to provide proof of this income, their costs for child care, or when their child was last covered by health insurance.

A major problem with programs for low-income children is that the low level of provider reimbursement has resulted in limited participation by doctors. This makes it difficult for parents to find a doctor who will accept this "insurance."

Every state has a program designed to offer wellness visits, vaccinations, and other care to children. But what is the biggest problem with these programs? Most parents and guardians don't know about them and don't know they probably qualify even if they have jobs.

You'll need the following to apply for these programs:

- ◆ Your family's most recent tax return (Form 1040)

- ◆ Your Wage and Earning Statement (W-2 Form)

- ◆ Current pay stubs covering the last 4 weeks

- ◆ The cost to add your child or children to health insurance coverage if your employer offers it

- ◆ Your child's Social Security number or the date applied for if you have not received a Social Security card

Call 1-877-KIDS NOW to get started.

The Least You Need to Know

- ◆ All states have programs designed to help children with uninsured parents get vaccines, have well-child visits, and see a doctor when they are sick.

- ◆ All children should see a pediatrician for vaccines, as well as for well-child visits and check-ups.

- ◆ Newborns must see a doctor regularly, beginning at two weeks and continuing every month or so until their first birthday; if you don't have insurance, call your local hospital to find out if it has a pediatrician who will help you.

- ◆ Children also need dental and vision care; ask your pediatrician or local pharmacy for offices that help uninsured kids get the care they need.

8

Health Care for People Ages 50–65

In This Chapter

◆ The importance of preventative care

◆ Medical tests and screenings

◆ Living a healthy lifestyle

◆ Participating in clinical trials

L'chaim! This is the Hebrew word Jewish people use when they make a toast, and it means "To life." These days, most of us live a long life, but how healthy we are later in life is very much a product of how we live. To a significant degree, the state of our health is up to us; Lifestyle choices, such as not smoking, eating well, and exercising, are huge predictors of how well we will age.

Of course, nothing can substitute for good genes. We can't do anything about your genetic material, but we can help you find ways to get good preventative care at a low cost.

Wellness Visits

You feel fine, right? So why should you, a person with no insurance, spend money on a doctor's visit? There may be a lot of reasons.

Although we have no statistics on how many people could avoid the emergency room and more expensive and invasive treatments by early detection of all diseases and illnesses, it is certainly true that the most serious conditions that kill Americans, such as heart disease and cancer (including skin, prostate, breast, and lung) are detectable by physicians during routine visits. For example, if everyone age 50 or older had regular screening tests, at least one-third of the deaths from these cancers could be avoided, according to the American Cancer Society.

For Your Health _____

Even as an adult, you need to stay up-to-date with your immunizations. According to the American Medical Association, you should have a flu shot every year starting at age 50. If you are younger than 50, ask your doctor whether you need a flu shot. Have a pneumonia shot once after you turn 65. If you are younger, ask your doctor whether you need a pneumonia shot. And be sure your doctor knows which other shots, such as tetanus, you need to keep up-to-date.

In fact, often, physicians simply have to ask questions or look you over. That new, mysterious mole, for example, might warrant a referral for further testing.

Now, if you don't have insurance, then you might simply set aside about $200 each year to see a doctor for preventive care.

Why $200? Chances are, unless you live in a major city, you can offer a doctor $100 or so in cash to see you for a check-up. You'll need the other $100 for tests, including blood tests and other work-ups for your specific sex and concerns.

And it's better for your health to have a relationship with a physician who will see you regularly and keep your records than to bounce around from one doctor to another because a doctor will notice changes in your body (such as moles) and will be more likely to see you in case of emergency.

Bet You Didn't Know

When employers first began offering health insurance in the 1940s, they didn't worry about long-term care for retirees because most people retired at or near 65 and life expectancy after that was about 12 years. Geriatric medicine was unknown, and there were no treatments for many of the diseases affecting the elderly.

Minimum Required Screenings and Immunizations

Here are the minimum required screenings and immunizations, according to the U.S. Department of Health and Human Services (HHS) and the United States Preventive Services Task Force.

For Your Health _____

Many emergency rooms and hospitals have Outpatient Offices, where you can get nonemergency care at a reduced rate. Call your local hospital to ask about getting any of the tests described in the following sections. If they can't help you, they will probably know where you can go. Simply say you don't have insurance, and tell them which test you want to have.

Body Mass Index Calculation

Obesity, how much fat is on your body, is a good indication of the state of your health as it is directly related to your risk of heart disease as well as other illnesses. You can do this yourself by going to www. nhlbisupport.com/bmi. You'll need to know your height and weight. But, of course, most of us know just by looking in the mirror if we need to lose weight!

High Cholesterol

This is done with a blood test and costs about $10 for a simple screening test and $50 for a complete lipid profile at a commercial (i.e., nonhospital) lab. Very often, however, you will see signs for Free Cholesterol Screenings at health fairs, hospitals, and pharmacies. Or call an American Heart Association office near you (they are in the phone book) to find out when they are holding free screenings.

Blood Pressure

Many pharmacies, gyms, and YMCAs have free blood pressure checks. A nurse can easily do this. Simply call a lab or doctor's office, and ask if you can have someone check this for you. They will most likely not charge you if you ask for a free screening blood pressure check or tell them you do not have insurance. Or call an American Heart Association office to find out when it is holding free screenings.

For Your Health

Blood pressure and life expectancy are directly proportional. The graph is a nearly straight line. The lower your blood pressure (down to about 100/60—below that you may not be able to stand up), the longer your life.

You can even buy an inexpensive stethoscope and sphygmomanometer (the blood pressure cuff and machine), or even a completely automatic blood pressure cuff, and ask your doctor or nurse to teach you how to use it. This is especially helpful if you are on medication for hypertension.

How high is "high" blood pressure? Blood pressure higher than 140/90 should be checked by a doctor. In fact, the American Heart Association recently changed the guidelines. So, you need to ask a doctor, or as we suggested, go to a local Heart Association office and talk to a physician there).

Colorectal Cancer

Have a test for colorectal cancer starting at age 50. If there is a family history of colorectal cancer, you may need to be screened earlier. Screening can find polyps, so they can be removed before they turn into cancer. For most adults, periodic colonoscopy (every 2–10 years based on your risk) is the screening test of choice. There are X-ray (virtual colonoscopy) techniques for this, but then if they spot a polyp you have to have the colonoscopy anyway. The X-ray tests may be good for someone who wants to avoid the procedure unless absolutely necessary, but the "bowel prep" is the same. For more information go to www.cdc.gov/cancer/screenforlife.

Diabetes

Screening for diabetes is done by measuring blood glucose or sugar. Many hospitals and clinics have free screenings, or you can go to the American Diabetes Association at www.defeatdiabetes.org to take an online screening test, which, if you score high, could indicate that you should have a blood test.

Depression (and Other Mental Health Issues)

Your emotional health is as important as your physical health. If you have felt down, sad, or hopeless over the last two weeks or have felt little interest or pleasure in doing things, you may be depressed. Call a local hospital to see if they have mental health screenings or if there is a local clinic who helps those with a mental illness. See Chapter 9 for more information.

Sexually Transmitted Diseases, Including HIV

People in their 50s could be at risk for sexually transmitted diseases if they are dating, especially if they were previously in monogamous relationships and aren't used to protecting themselves for these possibilities. A person of any age can get an STD. Talk to your doctor to see whether you should be tested for gonorrhea, syphilis, Chlamydia, or other sexually transmitted infections. Ask your doctor about HIV screening if you have had sex with men; have had unprotected sex with multiple partners; have used or now use injection drugs; exchange sex for money or drugs or have sex partners who do; have past or present sex partners who are HIV-infected, are bisexual, use injection drugs, or are being treated for sexually transmitted diseases.

The Wellness Life

Yes, you need to see a doctor periodically for preventive exams, and yes, you need to get the right tests and screenings to benefit from the knowledge of a doctor, but there is really no substitute for taking care of yourself.

Quit Smoking

The absolute most important thing you can do to take care of yourself is to quit smoking. Smoking causes both heart disease and cancer (the #1 and #2 killers in this country) as well as emphysema (which not only kills but makes what life you have left miserable), and a variety of vascular-related disease. It also causes wrinkles and makes you look old. Go to www.smokefree.gov or call the National Quitline (1-800-QUITNOW) for help. You can use the money you spent on cigarettes to save for seeing a doctor.

For Your Health

Ask your doctor about taking aspirin to prevent heart disease if you are older than 45 or younger than 45 and have high blood pressure, high cholesterol, diabetes, or you smoke.

By the way, smoking marijuana is even worse than smoking cigarettes because of all the inhaled debris and the increased length and depth of inhalation.

Join a Gym

Find some way to get regular (at least three to four times a week) exercise. Exercising will help you stay healthy in a number of ways. First, exercise helps fight age-related weight gain; it improves people's moods; and it fights weight-related diseases, such as diabetes and cardiovascular problems. If done right, exercise can keep your heart and other muscles in the best possible condition. Ask your doctor or a trainer at the gym for an exercise prescription.

There's another way gyms can help you stay healthy—they often have clinics and meetings featuring doctors, nurses, and other health expert from the community.

Gyms are generally thought of as expensive, but most towns have local YMCAs which offer reduced-rate memberships to local citizens. You may have to show them your financial statements, and you may not get a full discount, but the membership will pay for itself in terms of its health benefits.

But here's another idea: if you're out of work or can't afford a member-ship, ask if you can either volunteer or work at the gym in exchange for a membership. We know a woman who couldn't find an administrative job in her hometown, and the stress got to her so much, she went to the gym to find out about its rates. She ended up running the front desk, which didn't pay much, but it did get her a membership; and then, a few months later, she started to work as a personal trainer. Ten months later, she got the job she had originally wanted, but in the meantime she had created a second career and begun to make pretty good money. More than anything, the work paid off in building her self-confidence and allowing her to meet people.

For Your Health

If joining a gym doesn't work, you can start your own personal exer-cise program by adding activity into your life. Mowing the lawn, dancing, swimming, gardening, and bicycling are just a few exam-ples of beneficial physical activity. Start small and work up to 30 minutes or more of moderate physical activity most days (at least three) of the week. Whatever you do, try to make it enjoyable and a part of your regular routine.

Eat a Healthy Diet

Your diet should include fresh fruits, vegetables, whole grains, and fat-free or low-fat milk and milk products; include lean meats, poultry, fish, beans, eggs, and nuts. Try to avoid foods high in saturated fats, trans fats, cholesterol, salt (sodium), and added sugars. Unfortunately, Ameri-cans are currently in the throes of an obesity epidemic. There are many causes; fast foods, fried foods, highly processed foods, high-fat foods, large portions, and foods high in salt all contribute to the problem.

How much we eat is as important as what we eat. It is quite possible to become obese while eating "healthy" food if you eat too much of it. Portion sizes have grown over the years, along with our waistlines.

Obesity increases your risk of diabetes, hypertension, high cholesterol, heart disease, and cancer. Carrying extra weight overtaxes every organ in your body and stresses your joints, such as the hips and knees.

Drink Alcohol Only in Moderation

If you drink alcohol, have no more than two drinks a day. A standard drink is one 12-ounce bottle of beer or wine cooler, one 5-ounce glass of wine, or 1.5 ounces of 80-proof distilled spirits. Women should drink proportionately less due to their (generally) lower body mass. Alcohol also contains empty calories (7 calories per gram). Overindulgence in alcohol puts you at increased risk for cancer and accidents of all types.

Do Your Best to Avoid Accidents

Careful attention to safety when you drive, work, exercise, and even stay at home (slipping in the tub hurts thousands of people each year) can pay off in huge health benefits and financial savings over time. Accidents are usually foreseeable and preventable. Wear your seatbelt tight across your hips, not on top of your abdomen. Wear a helmet when you bicycle, and don't ride or run in heavy traffic. Think about safety as part of your everyday routine.

Maintain Contact With Your Friends

Love and support can go a long way, especially if you feel bad for struggling with an issue such as not having insurance or enough money to pay for the medical care you need. But having friends is good for your health. It helps your mood and is good for your heart (literally) and your soul.

Volunteer

You're struggling with what you don't have, money, insurance, but chances are you still have something to give, your time and energy. People who volunteer are healthier than those who don't.

Support Groups

Finding people to talk with does not in any way replace medical attention, but discussing your health issues with people who also suffer from the same problem is a way to both reduce stress and find possible solutions that you didn't know about.

We looked in our local newspaper (in a town of 30,000 surrounded by four towns of 10,000 people or fewer) and found support groups for overeating, macular degeneration, multiple sclerosis, smoking cessation, and melanoma. And if you don't find a support group for the health concern that troubles you, consider starting one. Maybe someone needs your support as much as you need theirs.

Discount Plans

There are many alternatives to traditional health insurance and Medicaid which might offer a discount on your health care and help you out. Check with your health care provider to find out what discount you would receive if you paid cash. Take monthly fees, deductibles, and premiums into account.

Code Red

Dozens of companies sell fake health-insurance plans, calling them association plans and discount health cards. The sales pitch features medical, dental, and prescription benefits with no exclusions or limitations. But usually the truth is that no health-care provider will accept the card because the company network doesn't actually exist. To avoid getting scammed, call your state department of insurance to see if the plan and the agent are licensed. If not, tear up the contract and report them. If the company or agent won't give you a list of providers until you sign the paperwork, don't sign and report the salesman.

Blood Donations

Donating blood was once a traditional way to earn money for medical students, college students, alcoholics, drug addicts, and others. But since the HIV/AIDS epidemic began, standards have tightened up significantly; you can no longer get money for this, and you also do not get results from a blood test.

If you give blood, you'll get a glass of juice but no real health care. Most donation centers these days are looking for volunteer donors, so don't expect to get paid. Likewise, most donation centers do not release the results of HIV testing in order to prevent high-risk people from donating blood in order to get tested.

However, donating blood is a great way to help others and, remember, that's a good way to help your health!

To learn more about donating blood, go to www.bloodforlife.org.

Clinics

Clinics may be a good source of care for someone with limited resources. Realize there may be issues of continuity of care (but this may be an issue at a large group practice as well) and that clinics are sometimes a place of great transition. Many teaching hospitals have clinics staffed primarily by residents (doctors in training) who are only there for a year or two. On the other hand, these people may well be highly motivated to provide excellent care, interested in their patients, and not jaded by many years of seeing the same thing over and over. Many community clinics fill a real health care void in their service area.

Also free clinics in most counties provide service to those unable to pay. You generally must show need and that you are not eligible for Medicaid or other insurance.

To find a clinic, look in the phone book, call a doctor's office and ask if they know of one, or call the hospital. Also look online by going to a search engine and typing in the name of your county or town and free clinic, or ask a librarian to help you find one.

Many doctors have worked in free clinics, but they limit their participation because it doesn't pay them very well. However, many excellent retired as well as actively practicing physicians volunteer, so it's not as if you will get inferior care.

Some hospitals support free clinics as a community service, and some do it to keep nonpaying patients out of their emergency room. This is why you can call a hospital to find out about out-patient services, which will, in the long run, be less expensive than going to an emergency room.

Doctors traditionally have allowed a certain amount of charity care in their regular practices. This is becoming harder for them to do as third-party payers (insurers) cut the doctor's pay even while their overhead (expenses) continue to increase.

Local Pharmacies/Supermarkets

These days many stores, both drug stores and grocery stores, realize they can fill a void (and make a profit) by providing the types of health care people without insurance or who are underinsured need. This is a perfectly safe way to get vaccinations and, if the person staffing the store clinic is a doctor or nurse practitioner, the better off you'll be with any health advice they offer, but remember that pharmacists are, by law, unable to give medical advice or care.

One drug store chain, Walgreens, offers a mobile lab service, a customized bus staffed by professionals who give medical screenings for a reduced price. The tests include total cholesterol level, blood pressure, bone density, glucose level, and body mass index.

Once again, this doesn't replace medical care, but it is a beginning in helping you find out the status of your overall health.

Taking Part in a Medical Study

Adults can also get medical care and be in touch with health-care professionals by taking part in a medical study, which is more correctly called a clinical trial. Clinical trials are studies designed to help physicians and scientists understand how a specific medicine or treatment works and how well it works.

Many medical research studies will provide you with free (related) health care, medications, incidental expenses, and possibly even a small stipend if you participate. This might be a good option for you if you are unemployed or have a disease being studied. Be sure you understand the terms of the study and what they expect of you.

If the research you participate in is a comparison study, you may be given a placebo and won't be told whether you're getting the medical treatment or if you are in the control group. This often applies to clinical trials sought after by cancer patients.

Drug companies and government safety boards, as well as hospitals and other researchers, use clinical trials to determine if a specific treatment should become part of standard treatment.

There are always three to four phases in a clinical trial, and you do not have to take part in all phases. The early phases make sure the treatment is safe. Later phases show if what is being tested (a drug, a life-style change, a medical protocol) works better than the standard treatment.

Clinical Trial Phase	Number of People Needed	Purpose
Phase I	15-30 people	To find a safe dose; to decide how the new treatment should be given; to see how the new treatment affects the human body
Phase II	Less than 100 people	To determine if the new treatment has an effect on a certain disease; to see how the new treatment affects the human body
Phase III	From 100 to thousands of people	To compare the new treatment (or new use of a treatment) with the current standard treatment
Phase IV	Several hundred to several thousand people	To further assess the long-term safety and effectiveness of a new treatment

No matter what organization is doing the research, all clinical trials clearly state who will be able to join the study and the treatment plan. Every trial has a person in charge, usually a doctor, who is called the principal investigator. The principal investigator prepares a plan for the study, called a *protocol*, which is like a recipe for conducting a clinical trial.

Most participants in a clinical trial will need to be screened to see if they are an appropriate candidate for the study. Based on the questions the research is trying to answer, each clinical trial protocol clearly states who can or cannot join the trial.

def•i•ni•tion

The **protocol** explains what the trial will do, how the study will be carried out, and why each part of the study is necessary. It includes why the study is being done; who can join the study; how many people are needed for the study; what if any drugs they will take, the dose, and how often; what medical tests they will have and how often; and what information will be gathered about them.

For example, sometimes researchers are looking for people who have a certain disease or symptom, who have received a certain kind of therapy in the past, who are a specific age or sex, or who are at risk for specific illnesses.

If you are interested in joining a trial, you will receive medical tests to be sure that you are not put at increased risk.

By looking at the pros and cons of clinical trials and your other treatment choices, you are taking an active role in a decision that affects your life. You have the chance to help others and improve their health care. However, clinical trials are not for everyone. New treatments under study are not always better than, or even as good as, standard care.

Bet You Didn't Know

Federal laws help insure that all clinical trials are run in an ethical manner. Your rights and safety are protected through informed consent, and careful review and approval of the clinical trial protocol is inspected by two review panels, including a scientific review panel and an institutional review board (IRB), as well as the care of the research team.

Likewise, new treatments may have side effects that doctors do not expect or that are worse than those of standard treatment. Similarly, even if a new treatment has benefits, it may not work for you. Even standard treatments, proven effective for many people, do not help everyone.

If you want to take part in a clinical trial, consider these questions:

◆ Why is this trial being done?

◆ How long will I be in the trial?

- Why do the doctors who designed the trial believe that the treatment being studied may be better than the one being used now? Why may it not be better?

- What kinds of tests and treatments are involved?

- What are the possible side effects or risks of the new treatment?

- What are the possible benefits?

- How will the doctor know if the treatment is working?

- Will I have to pay for any of the treatments or tests?

- What costs will my health insurance cover?

- How could the trial affect my daily life?

- How often will I have to come to the hospital or clinic?

- Will I have to travel long distances?

- What are my other treatment choices, including standard treatments?

- How does the treatment I would receive in this trial compare with the other treatment choices?

Some trials offer stipends to those who take part, especially if the study involves time away from your home, such as sleeping at a sleep clinic.

The National Cancer Institute, drug companies, medical institutions, and other organizations sponsor clinical trials. These trials take place in many settings, such as cancer centers, large medical centers, small hospitals, and doctors' offices. To find out about all types of trails go to www.clinicaltrials.gov. Also go to local colleges and hospitals to find out about studies taking place in your area, since college students and those already in the medical system are often willing to take part in this very important work.

Insurance Issues

Most of us like to believe that our financial security, including our health insurance status, increases as we get older. But unfortunately, that isn't always the case. According to The Center on an Aging Society based at Georgetown University, a large population of adults aged 55 to 65 have little or no insurance but struggle with a chronic condition, such as asthma, diabetes, or cardiovascular disease.

Of those Americans with chronic conditions, 66 percent have private insurance either through their employer or their own policy, while 22 percent have public insurance, such as through Medicaid, Medicare, or a combination, and 12 percent—about 1.5 million Americans—have no health insurance.

> **Bet You Didn't Know**
>
> Over half of all adults age 55 to 65 (that's 13 million Americans) have arthritis, cancer, diabetes, heart disease, or hypertension.

But the numbers regarding the insured and the uninsured do not tell the whole story. Because many employers are cutting down on their contribution to insurance, older Americans, who are far more likely than younger Americans to have a chronic illness, spend twice as much for health care as younger adults.

This problem of rising out-of-pocket health-care costs combined with health issues has made saving for retirement—and having a healthy retirement—difficult for older Americans.

According to the Commonwealth Fund:

◆ High blood pressure, arthritis, and high cholesterol are the most common health problems facing older Americans, and 62 percent of 50–64 year-olds in working households report having at least one chronic illness.

◆ Those with the lowest incomes—but who are working—report that they have no means to get insurance because they can't afford private coverage but are ineligible for public insurance.

◆ More than half of older Americans with private coverage spend more than $300 per month ($3,600 annually) on health insurance. Three out of five of those adults say it is difficult for them to pay for this coverage.

◆ Despite high premiums, this group of Americans also has high deductibles, often close to or above $1,000.

About three-quarters of Americans think Medicare should be expanded and that same number also want to find a way to put savings toward their long-term health care through a pretax, out-of-their-paycheck program.

These adults understand that Medicare will not cover all of their medical expenses as they get older.

The Least You Need to Know

◆ No matter what your financial or insurance status, try to see a doctor periodically (depending on your age, sex, and risk factors) for basic medical tests and preventive care, which, in the end, could save your health and cost you less money than more intensive medical treatment.

◆ There are low-cost ways to get basic preventive medical care, such as vaccines, which adults need, too, and screenings.

◆ Live healthfully to reduce your need to visit doctors for illness.

◆ Clinical trials and other medical studies can provide good health care, as well as some money, to all types of patients.

Chapter 9

Mental Health Care

In This Chapter

- ◆ Symptoms and diagnostic care
- ◆ Physicians and referrals
- ◆ Talking to the right person
- ◆ Addiction counseling

According to the American Psychological Association, mental health disorders affect people from childhood to old age, both men and women, in all regions of the country, and individuals of all socioeconomic groups. Each year, 1 in 10 Americans experiences some disability from a mental health disorder.

Fortunately psychological research and a variety of therapies and medications have improved the diagnosis and treatment of mental health disorders. Today, many of these disorders are preventable, controllable, or curable.

Right now, the American Psychological Association estimates that 15 to 18 percent of Americans, including nearly 10 million children, suffer from a diagnosable mental disorder. And because the mind also affects the body, 50 to 70 percent of visits to primary care physicians are for medical complaints that stem from psychological factors.

Physically ill and older people are more likely to suffer from mental health disorders. More than half of Americans 65 years and older who are treated for physical illness in hospitals, clinics, and nursing homes also have at least one identifiable mental health problem. And according to a study by the National Institute of Mental Health (NIMH), separated or divorced people are twice as likely as married people to have a mental health disorder.

> **For Your Health**
>
> Mental health treatment typically means some form of therapy, such as talking with a therapist, as well as the use of medication.

Also unfortunately, poorer people are consistently more likely to have a mental health disorder than people who are socially and financially better off.

> **Bet You Didn't Know**
>
> Medical complaints arise from psychological factors at least as often as they do from physical problems. Also mental health disorders, particularly depression and anxiety, often aggravate physical illnesses, especially in older people.

Combination of Therapies

Getting an accurate diagnosis is most important, so you can get the right treatment for your condition.

When you look for mental health care, you have the option of speaking with a variety of health care professionals, including:

◆ a clinical psychologist, a professional with a doctoral degree in psychology who specializes in therapy.

◆ a psychiatrist, a professional who completed both medical school and training in psychiatry and is a specialist in diagnosing and treating mental illness.

- a clinical social worker, a professional with an advanced degree in social work who provides services for the prevention, diagnosis, and treatment of mental and behavioral disorders.

- a registered nurse, a trained professional with a nursing degree who provides patient care and administers medicine.

- a nurse practitioner, a registered nurse who works in an expanded role and manages patients' medical conditions.

Any of these qualified practitioners is referred to as a specialist if he or she has received advanced education in a particular area of health care, such as mental illness or substance abuse.

For Your Health

American Psychological Association studies show that including mental health treatment as part of the overall treatment plan for people with certain physical illnesses, such as cancer and diabetes, can enhance recovery or halt progression of the disease, thereby using fewer medical resources.

Getting Care

Getting proper mental health care can be problematic. Many medical insurance plans have limited benefits for hospitalization and other types of mental health care. Many mental health providers limit the types of insurance they accept and some will not accept insurance at all. It pays to read the specifics in your policy to determine what level of coverage you have.

If you find yourself in need of mental health services it may make sense to start with a referral from your primary care physician. Ideally he will help you navigate through the maze of different practitioners and help select the most appropriate level and source of care. Many primary care physicians even consider basic mental health problems (such as depression) within their scope of practice and may be able to treat you themselves or in conjunction with a medical health professional.

In the absence of medial insurance your only option may be to pay out of pocket, or to go to the local public health mental health clinic. These are funded on a state by state basis (see below) and vary widely in terms of access, waiting times, and the level of service available.

Other therapeutic options include:

◆ Community mental health centers (CMHCs). These centers offer a range of mental health treatment and counseling services, usually at a reduced rate for low-income people. CMHCs often require you to have a private insurance plan or to be a recipient of public assistance.

◆ Pastoral counseling. Your church or synagogue can put you in touch with a pastoral counseling program. Certified pastoral counselors, who are ministers in a recognized religious body, have advanced degrees in pastoral counseling, as well as professional counseling experience. Pastoral counseling is often provided on a sliding-scale fee basis.

◆ Self-help groups. Another option is to join a self-help or support group. Such groups give people a chance to learn about, talk about, and work on their common problems, such as alcoholism, substance abuse, depression, family issues, and relationships. Self-help groups are generally free and can be found in virtually every community in America. Many people find them to be effective.

◆ Public assistance. People with severe mental illness may be eligible for several forms of public assistance, both to meet the basic costs of living and to pay for health care. Examples of such programs are Social Security, Medicare, and Medicaid.

Social Security has two types of programs to help individuals with disabilities. Social Security Disability Insurance provides benefits for those individuals who have worked for a required length of time and have paid Social Security taxes. Supplemental Security Income provides benefits to individuals based on their economic needs (Social Security Administration, 2002).

For information about Medicaid, contact your local social service or welfare office. You can also find information about Medicare and Medicaid at www.CMS.gov.

For information about Community Mental Health Centers, contact:

National Council for Community Behavioral Health Care
12300 Twinbrook Parkway, Suite 320
Rockville, MD 20852

Telephone: 301-984-6200
Fax: 301-881-7159
www.nccbh.org

> ### Bet You Didn't Know
>
> Most therapists who work in a one-on-one setting with an individual are licensed social workers. Look for M.S.W. or L.S.W. after their name.

Mental Health Medication

According to a new study in the journal *Health Affairs*, treatment for mental illness is a major driver of health care inflation and second only to heart disease. And among mental health treatments, the study concludes that antidepressant drugs known as SSRIs are a big contributor to that cost inflation. Over the last year, pharmacies filled more than $146 million in prescriptions for SSRIs.

These growing costs have led many employers to view mental health benefits as a potential drain on profits, making businesses reluctant to provide health insurance coverage for mental illness.

 Code Red

> Do not mistake talking to friends as a substitute for therapy. It's not. While friends may love you and be helpful, they cannot be responsible for your mental health.

Substance Abuse Treatment

The Substance Abuse and Mental Health Services Administration (SAMHSA) works to encourage experts and hospitals to help individuals building resilience for a successful recovery from addiction.

There is a distinct difference in spending trends between public and private organizations that pay for substance abuse treatment. During a long-term study done by SAMSHA, on average, private insurance payments for substance abuse treatment fell 1.6 percent each year during the study period while public sector expenditures increased 7.5 percent each year.

In 1986, private insurance paid $2.8 billion for drug and alcohol treatment; by 2003, it funded $2.1 billion in treatment—a 24 percent decline. The share of total substance abuse treatment costs paid by private insurance declined from 30 percent to 10 percent. Medicaid and other public sources contributed 50 percent of substance abuse treatment costs in the United States in 1986. Their portion climbed to 77 percent by 2003.

In fact, states pay the largest share of mental health and substance abuse treatment (you'll notice that every state listed in this chapter has a department of mental health). In 1998, Medicaid and other state and local agencies covered 39 percent of the total cost of drug and alcohol treatment. By 2003, their share grew to 58 percent.

According to Thomson Healthcare, about 22.5 million Americans suffer from a substance use disorder in any given year, and less than 4 million receive treatment. Ironically, though, because an overwhelming percentage of people with substance abuse problems do not have health insurance, there are often more public programs for these issues than there are for other health issues, such as dental and vision care.

To find substance abuse treatment in your state, look for phone numbers and websites below, but be warned, to find the right program for you or a loved one, you will probably need to do a lot more research than just dialing these numbers. As always, ask lots of questions about the care you are entitled to and be sure to keep records of whom you speak with.

- ◆ Alabama: Substance Abuse Services Division. Call 334-242-3961, or go to www.mh.alabama.gov.

- ◆ Alaska: Health and Social Services. Call 1-877-266-4357, or go to www.hss.state.ak.us/dbh.

- ◆ Arizona: Department of Health Services. Call 602-364-4558, or go to www.azdhs.gov.

- ◆ Arkansas: Office of Alcohol & Drug Abuse Prevention. Call 501-686-9866, or go to www.ardhs.sharepointsite.net/ARSOC/default.aspx.

- ◆ California: Alcohol and Drug Abuse Division. Call 1-800-879-2772, or go to www.adp.ca.gov.

- ◆ Colorado: Alcohol and Drug Abuse Division. Call 303-866-7480, or go to www.cdhs.state.co.us/adad.

◆ Connecticut: Department of Mental Health and Addiction Services. Call 860-418-6962, or go to www.ct.gov/dmhas/site/default.asp.

◆ Delaware: Alcohol and Drug Services, Division of Substance Abuse and Mental Health. Call 302-255-9399, or go to www.dhss. delaware.gov/dsamh/index.html.

◆ District of Columbia: Addiction, Prevention, and Recovery Administration. Call 202-727-8857, or go to www.dchealth.dc. gov/doh/cwp/view,a,3,Q,573170.asp.

◆ Florida: Substance Abuse Program Office, Florida Dept of Children & Families. Call 850-487-2920, or go to www.dcf.state. fl.us/mentalhealth/sa.

◆ Georgia: Addictive Diseases Program. Call 404-657-2275, or go to www.mhddad.dhr.georgia.gov/portal/site/dhr-mhddad.

◆ Hawaii: Alcohol and Drug Abuse Division. Call 808-692-7506, or go to www.hawaii.gov/health/substance-abuse.

◆ Idaho: Division of Behavioral Health, Department of Health & Welfare. Call 208-334-5935, or go to www.healthandwelfare.idaho. gov/site/3460/default.aspx.

◆ Illinois: Division of Alcoholism and Substance Abuse, Department of Human Services. Call 312-814-3840, or go to www.dhs.state. il.us/oasa.

◆ Indiana: Division of Mental Health and Addiction Family and Social Services Administration. Call 317-232-7800, or go to www. in.gov/fssa/mental.

◆ Iowa: Bureau of Substance Abuse and Prevention, Department of Public Health. Call 515-281-4417, or go to www.idph.state.ia.us/ bh/substance_abuse.asp.

◆ Kansas: Social and Rehabilitation Services. Call 785-291-3326, or go to www.srskansas.org/accesspoints/substance.htm.

◆ Kentucky: Division of Mental Health & Substance Abuse. Call 502-564-2880, or go to www.mhmr.ky.gov/mhsas.

◆ Louisiana: Office for Addictive Disorders, Department of Health and Hospitals. Call 225-342-6717, or go to www.dhh.louisiana. gov/offices/?ID=23.

For Your Health _____

Mental health hotlines and suicide prevention lines can help you even if you aren't in an emergency situation. Call them for help finding a doctor as well as substance abuse meetings and information. The numbers are usually in the phone book, or call the operator, information, or the police.

◆ Maine: Office of Substance Abuse, Department of Health and Human Services. Call 207-287-2595, or go to www.maine. gov/dhhs/osa.

◆ Maryland: Alcohol and Drug Abuse Administration, Department of Health and Mental Hygiene. Call 410-402-8600, or go to www. maryland-adaa.org/ka/index.cfm.

◆ Massachusetts: Bureau of Substance Abuse Services, Department of Public Health. Call 617-624-5111, or go to www.mass.gov and search under substance abuse.

◆ Michigan: Office of Drug Control Policy, Bureau of Substance Abuse & Addiction Services. Call 1-888-736-0253 or go to www. michigan.gov/mdch/0,1607,7-132-2941_4871---,00.html.

◆ Minnesota: Chemical Health Division, Department of Human Services. Call 651-431-2460, or go to www.dhs.state.mn.us and search under mental health or substance abuse.

◆ Mississippi: Division of Alcohol & Drug Abuse, Department of Mental Health. Call 601-359-1288, or go to www.dmh.state.ms. us/substance_abuse_services.html.

◆ Missouri: Division of Alcohol and Drug Abuse, Missouri Department of Mental Health. Call 573-751-4942, or go to www.dmh. missouri.gov/ada/adaindex.htm.

◆ Montana: Addictive & Mental Disorders Division, Department of Public Health and Human Services. Call 406-444-3964, or go to www.dphhs.mt.gov/index.shtml.

◆ Nebraska: Division of Behavioral Health Services Department of Health & Human Services Systems. Call 402-471-7818, or go to www.hhss.ne.gov/sua/suaindex.htm.

◆ Nevada: Substance Abuse Prevention & Treatment Agency. Call 775-684-4190, or go to mhds.state.nv.us.

◆ New Hampshire: Office of Alcohol and Drug Policy. Call 603-271-6110, or go to www.dhhs.nh.gov/DHHS/Programs+Services/default.htm.

◆ New Jersey: Division of Addiction Services. Call 609-292-5760, or go to www.state.nj.us/humanservices/das/index.htm.

◆ New Mexico: Behavioral Health Services Division, Human Services Department. Call 505-827-2601, or go to www.hsd.state.nm.us/bhsd.

◆ New York: Office Of Alcoholism and Substance Abuse Services. Call 518-485-1768, or go to www.oasas.state.ny.us/index.cfm.

◆ North Carolina: Community Policy Management, Division of Mental Health, Developmental Disabilities, and Substance Abuse Services. Call 919-733-4670, or go to www.dhhs.state.nc.us/mhddsas.

◆ North Dakota: Department of Human Services. Call 701-328-8920, or go to www.nd.gov/dhs/services/mentalhealth.

◆ Ohio: Department of Alcohol and Drug Addiction Services. Call 614-466-3445, or go to www.ada.ohio.gov/GD/Templates/Pages/ODADAS/ODADASDefault.aspx?page=1.

◆ Oklahoma: Department of Mental Health & Substance Abuse Services. Call 405-522-3619, or go to www.odmhsas.org.

◆ Oregon: Addictions & Mental Health Division, Department of Human Services. Call 503-945-5763, or go to www.oregon.gov/DHS/addiction/index.shtml.

◆ Pennsylvania: Bureau of Drug and Alcohol Programs. Call 717-783-8200, or go to www.health.state.pa.us/bdap.

◆ Rhode Island: Behavioral Health Care, Division of Behavioral Health, Department of Mental Health & Retardation. Call 401-462-4680, or go to www.mhrh.ri.gov/SA.

◆ South Carolina: Department of Alcohol and Other Drug Abuse Services. Call 803-896-5555, or go to www.daodas.state.sc.us.

- South Dakota: Division of Alcohol and Drug Abuse, Department of Human Services. Call 605-773-3123, or go to www.dhs.sd.gov.

- Tennessee: Department of Mental Health, Tennessee Department of Health. Call 615-741-1921, or go to www.health.state.tn. us/index.shtml.

- Texas: Mental Health and Substance Abuse, Department of State Health Services. Call 512-206-5000, or go to www.dshs.state. tx.us/mentalhealth.shtm.

- Utah: Division of Substance Abuse and Mental Health. Call 801-538-3939, or go to www.dsamh.utah.gov.

- Vermont: Division of Alcohol and Drug Abuse Programs, Department of Health. Call 802-651-1550, or go to www.healthvermont. gov/mh/index.aspx.

- Virginia: Office of Substance Abuse Services Dept. of MH, MR, & SAS. Call 804-786-3906, or go to www.dmhmrsas.virginia.gov.

- Washington: Div of Alcohol and Substance Abuse Dept of Social and Health Services. Call 1-877-301-4557, or go to www1.dshs. wa.gov/DASA.

- West Virginia: Division on Alcoholism and Drug Abuse, Office of Behavioral Health Services. Call 304-558-2276, or go to www. wvdhhr.org/bhhf/ada.asp.

- Wisconsin: Bureau of Mental Health and Substance Abuse Services. Call 608-266-2717, or go to www.dhfs.state.wi. us/substabuse/index.htm.

- Wyoming: Substance Abuse Division, Department of Health. Call 307-777-3353, or go to www.wdh.state.wy.us/mhsa/index.html.

Other important numbers:

- SAMHSA's National Mental Health Information Center, P.O. Box 42557, Washington, D.C. 20015; 1-800-789-2647; www. mentalhealth.samhsa.gov.

- Centers for Medicare and Medicaid Services, 7500 Security Boulevard, Baltimore, MD 21244-1850; 1-877-267-2323; www.cms.gov.

◆ National Mental Health Consumers' Self-Help Clearinghouse, 1211 Chestnut Street, Suite 1207, Philadelphia, PA 19107; 1-800-553-4539.

For more information about how to pay for mental health care, consider the following:

National Mental Health Information Center
P.O. Box 42557
Washington, D.C. 20015
1-800-789-2647
www.mentalhealth.samhsa.gov

American Association of Pastoral Counselors
9504-A Lee Highway
Fairfax, VA 22031-2303
703-385-6967
www.aapc.org

American Self-Help Clearinghouse
Saint Clare's Hospital
100 E. Hanover Avenue
Cedar Knolls, NJ 07927
973-326-8853
www.mentalhelp.net/selfhelp

National Alliance for the Mentally Ill
Colonial Place Three
2107 Wilson Boulevard, Suite 300
Arlington, VA 22201-3042
1-800-950-6264
www.nami.org

National Empowerment Center
599 Canal Street
Lawrence, MA 01840
1-800-769-3728
www.power2u.org

National Mental Health Consumer's Self-Help Clearinghouse
1211 Chestnut Street, Suite 1207
Philadelphia, PA 19107
1-800-553-4539
www.mhselfhelp.org

The Least You Need to Know

◆ Getting the right diagnosis for an emotional problem is always crucial, so see a therapist or psychiatrist, even if you have to pay out of pocket, and take some time to sort through your feelings.

◆ If you are in a crisis situation, call a hotline and be honest; tell them how you feel so they can help you.

◆ Find out if you can use a generic medication along with talk therapy.

◆ If you have a substance abuse problem, you may need to get public assistance for treatment if you are uninsured, unless you can pay for hospitalization out-of-pocket.

Chapter 10

Dental and Vision Care

In This Chapter

- ◆ Handling dental emergencies
- ◆ Preventative care
- ◆ Ongoing dental and vision care
- ◆ Insurance options for dental and vision care

In the ongoing political debates about health care, hardly anyone ever mentions teeth! It seems as if doctors, politicians, and even consumers consider straight, clean teeth and gums a luxury. Even health insurance companies don't include dental care in their medical policies. Of course, separating dental care from medical care might just be a way for them to collect another premium.

For a number of reasons, this attitude is problematic for Americans. First, far more Americans go without dental care than go without other medical care. But second, and far more important, dental health has been shown to be directly connected to other elements of health, including cardiovascular health.

Vision care is also a forgotten element of health care, even though, obviously, millions of Americans need glasses, contacts, and care for eye conditions, such as cataracts and glaucoma.

Finding and getting good dental and vision care isn't easy, but if you do research and develop a good relationship with the providers, you will have more luck in getting what you need at a reasonable cost.

Dental Emergencies

According to the American Dental Association, you should do these things for various dental emergencies before you contact a dentist for care:

Toothache

- Brush and rinse your teeth with warm water to keep them as clean as possible.

- Use dental floss to remove any trapped food between the teeth.

- Don't place an aspirin on the aching tooth or gum tissue.

Knocked-Out Tooth

- Rinse the tooth in running water if it's dirty.

- Don't scrub the tooth to clean it or remove any attached tissue fragments.

- Gently insert and hold the tooth in its socket or place it in a cup of milk or cool water.

- Go straight to a dentist or dental clinic. Very few emergency rooms have a dentist on call. If you get there within 30 minutes or less, there's a good chance the tooth can be put back into its proper place.

Broken Tooth

◆ Gently clean dirt from the injured area with warm water.

◆ Place a cold compress on the injured area to decrease swelling.

Severely Cut Tongue or Lip

◆ Apply direct pressure to the bleeding area with a clean cloth to stop the bleeding.

◆ Apply a cold compress to the injured area to decrease swelling and bleeding.

◆ Go to an emergency room if the bleeding doesn't stop.

Broken Jaw

◆ Try to keep your mouth and jaw still.

◆ Tie a handkerchief, necktie, or towel around the jaw and over the top of your head to keep your jaw in place and reduce movement.

◆ Apply a cold compress if swelling is present.

◆ Go to a hospital emergency room for further evaluation.

Dental care usually involves cleaning and preventive care, but it can sometimes mean dealing with toothaches or broken teeth and, rarely, a malignancy or tumor. Preventative dental care is important because gum disease is a serious illness that can have dangerous implications.

Bet You Didn't Know

For decades, the American Heart Association recommended that patients with certain heart conditions take antibiotics shortly before dental treatment. This was done with the belief that antibiotics would prevent infective endocarditis (IE), previously referred to as bacterial endocarditis. The AHA's latest guidelines were published in its scientific journal, *Circulation*, in April 2007 with good news; the AHA recommends that most of these patients no longer need short-term antibiotics as a preventive measure before their dental treatment.

Ongoing Dental Care

Like wellness visits and medical screens, you should see a dentist regularly. The American Dental Association recommends:

- Dental examinations—twice per year

- Bite-wing x-rays—once per year

- Teeth cleanings—twice per year

- Full mouth x-ray series—once every three years

Additionally, children and adolescents need more specific dental care, including topical fluoride treatments twice a year. Of course, your particular teeth may need more specialized and intensive dental care.

As with regular medical care, dentists accept payment in cash. You can use money from your health savings account (HSA) for dental care, or just put aside money for regular and emergency dental care. As in any cash transaction providers may be willing to negotiate on rates, accept credit cards, set up payment plans, or in other ways accommodate a patient.

Dental Insurance

If you have bad teeth or know you will need extensive dental care, you might look into buying dental insurance. This insurance exists to encourage members to get regular preventive dental care including checkups, cleanings, x-rays, sealants, and fluoride in order to prevent the more expensive treatments that come from poor dental habits.

> **For Your Health**
>
> If you are buying dental insurance, be sure to ask what happens during a dental emergency, especially one that may occur when you are out of town, possibly in an area where there are no provider dentists for the plan.

In fact, according to the American Dental Association, very few dental costs are caused by unpredictable events, such as an accident, but rather by situations where minor problems were not detected and dealt with within an appropriate time frame.

Dental insurance plan options are very similar to traditional health insurance in that you can get indemnity insurance, join a preferred provider network, or opt for a health maintenance type plan.

Dental Indemnity Plans

This is the conventional type of dental plan where you pay a monthly (or quarterly) premium as well as a co-payment when you see the dentist. These fees can range dramatically depending on where you live. According to the ADA, however, a typical indemnity plan reimburses at the rate of 100 percent for diagnostic and preventive treatment, 80 percent for routine operative treatment, extractions, root canals, and periodontal care, and 50 percent for major treatment like crowns, bridges, implants, and partial dentures up to the annual maximum. Indemnity plans may or may not cover *orthodontic* care, and if coverage is provided, there may be a lifetime maximum of $1,000, and orthodontia is often far more expensive than that.

def•i•ni•tion

An **orthodontist** corrects abnormally aligned or positioned teeth. Visit an orthodontist if problems associated with allergies or nasal obstructions are affecting your facial development or jawbone structure.

Most indemnity plans have many limitations and exclusions as to what benefits they will and will not pay for. Likewise, there is often an annual limit for care of any type, which can range from $1,000 to $2,500. Benefits are paid based on claims submitted for treatment done by the dentist with payment going to either the dentist or the employee. Most commonly, the dentist submits the claim for the patient with reimbursement directly to the dentist.

Bet You Didn't Know

According to the book *Uninsured in America*, by Harvard researchers Susan Starr Sered and Rushika Fernandopulle, most people without health insurance give up going to the dentist because of cost, and yet, at the same time, when these same people are asked what one thing bothers them most about their health and they first want to fix, it is their teeth.

As with medical insurance, some dental plans are self-funded, which means the organization who has contracted with the insurer underwrites the plan. In this case, you are typically reimbursed based on a schedule of funds allocated for care, rather than as a percentage of the cost of the type of treatment received.

So for example, the plan may reimburse 100 percent of the first $100 spent on care, 80 percent of the next $500, and 50 percent of the next $1,000 with an annual maximum of $1,000. If this is the case, the subscriber would have to pay out $600 as her share of the treatment costs before reaching the annual maximum. Another option of a self-funding plan is that 50 percent of the first $1,000 is paid by the organization, for a maximum annual benefit of $500.

> **For Your Health**
>
> Most dental insurance plans will not reimburse you for cosmetic procedures, such as bleaching or laser treatments to whiten your teeth.

Sometimes these plans are administered not by an insurance company but by the organization offering the plan or by a third party administrator.

> **For Your Health**
>
> The importance of brushing your teeth cannot be stressed enough. Take two to three minutes to brush your teeth, about the length of the average pop song. So listen to the radio or sing a song to yourself as you brush.

Managed Care Plans

More managed care plans are also available these days. In these plans, a dentist is contractually limited both by the types of treatment he can render to patients and also the fees that he can charge for that treatment.

With this type of plan, you must find a dentist within the network because this dentist has signed a contract with the insurance company agreeing to the limits on fees and treatment options.

Therefore, in these plans, patients may not be reimbursed for some of the various treatment options due to limitations in the plan. In addition, if you go out of the network, you will pay more money for treatment. While these costs are higher, the monthly premiums are typically less money than in other types of plans.

Preferred Provider Organization (PPO) plans

This type of plan, which is a type of managed care, includes both in-network and out-of-network dentists. Seeing an in-network dentist is less expensive, of course, but the premiums are the same each month.

Before you buy dental insurance, ask if dental specialists are included as service providers for the plan for those times when you might need the types of services they offer. Also ask if there are any restrictions on the amount of access you have to participating dentists and dental treatment. And find out if appointments are easily scheduled or if there is a lengthy waiting period.

Finally, realize that most dental insurance plans offer less coverage for higher-priced dental treatments including filings or restorative dental treatment, root canals or endodontic treatment, gum treatment or periodontal care, and tooth extractions and oral surgery.

The best place to find plans, providers, and other dental information is the website of the American Dental Association: www.ada.org.

Reduced-Cost Dental Programs

Many programs throughout the United States help people who struggle to pay their dental bills and who don't have dental insurance. In some cases, volunteers and nonprofit organizations run the programs, while others are part of state, county, or other local service departments.

Likewise, many dental schools offer appointments to people who are willing to be seen by a dental student or student dental hygienist. Contact a local dental school or university hospital to find out about these options.

While we can't go through every program throughout the country, especially since each program has its own mission as well as its own way of functioning, we can give you some ideas of what you might do to try to find a local program and what the majority of programs are able to offer its customers.

> ### Code Red
>
> It is very important to look for the ADA Seal of Acceptance on the box or label of all dental products you buy, especially since, in the summer of 2007, the U.S. Food and Drug Administration found the poisonous chemical diethylene glycol (DEG) in toothpaste imported from China. In fact, none of the toothpaste brands in the alert had received the Seal of Acceptance from the American Dental Association (ADA).

Getting Care

The great majority of reduced cost dental programs help children, seniors, and others who are less able to afford dental care, such as mentally or physically challenged people.

Before anyone can get care, though, he usually has to show he is a resident of the state or county offering the care. Once someone has brought in proof of residency, he will typically have to show proof of his limited resources, and then the organization will usually charge for the services provided based on income level.

So the question is, where can you find good dental care if you need help paying the bill? Well, first try calling your local city or county health department because they will typically know of any programs designed to help individuals get care.

> ### For Your Health
>
> If you or someone you know qualifies for special needs programs, contact The National Foundation of Dentistry for the Handicapped, 1800 15th St. #100, Denver, CO 80202; 303-534-5360, or go to www.nfdh.org/dds.html.

Or try going to the website of your state's dental association. In general, there are two types of dental organizations and dental websites. Some dental organizations and their websites are designed for dentists and have lots of information on how to get equipment and find a good malpractice lawyer! Those are not very helpful to you, the consumer!

But other dental organizations are filled with lots of helpful names and telephone numbers, as well as insurance and financial assistance programs for people who need it.

State-by-State Information

◆ Alabama: Call the Alabama Dental Association at 334-265-1684, or go to www.aldaonline.org.

◆ Alaska: A number of programs offer low-cost dental care, including The Community Health Centers and Donated Dental Services (DDS) which usually helps those with special needs. To find out more, call 907-248-3775. Medicaid covers adults for dental care, while children can use the Denali KidCare Program. Go to www.hss.state.ak.us/dhcs/denalikidscare, or call Denali KidCare at 1-888-318-8890.

◆ Arizona: Very little information about assistance for dental care is on the website, but call them for more information, especially if you want to get dental care for a child. Go to www.azda.org, or call 480-344-5777.

◆ Arkansas: Call the Arkansas State Dental Association for information at 501-834-7650, or go to www.dental-asda.org. Some organizations offer free dental care once a year.

◆ California: Reach the California Dental Association by calling 1-800-232-7645 or going to www.cda.org. Click on patient and community resources to learn more about your options.

◆ Colorado: Go to the Colorado Dental Association website at www.cdaonline.org, or call 303-740-6900. Information is given online about a direct reimbursement plan endorsed by the dental association.

◆ Connecticut: Reach the Connecticut Dental Association by calling 860-378-1800 or going to www.csda.com. The Connecticut Mission of Mercy sometimes offers free dental care or screenings in local communities.

◆ Delaware: Call 302-368-7634, or go to www.delawarestatedentalsociety.org/clinics.html to learn more about free clinics.

- District of Columbia: Reach the D.C. Dental Society at 202-547-7613, or go to www.dcdental.org.

- Florida: Call the Florida Dental Association at 850-681-3628, or go to www.floridadental.org to learn more about Pelican Dental Concepts, a self-funded dental plan. The FDA also sponsors statewide public-outreach programs, including Give Kids A Smile, which provides free dental care to underserved children. Also Dentists Care, an FDA charitable organization, seeks to serve underprivileged Floridians. E-mail fda@floridadental.org to learn more.

- Georgia: The Georgia Dental Association offers information for residents as well as dental care plans for those in the state insurance program. Call 404-636-7553, or go to www.gadental.org to learn more.

- Hawaii: Not a lot of information is on the website, www.hawaiidentalassociation.net, so if you live in Hawaii, to learn more about access to dental care, call 808-593-7956.

- Idaho: Reach the Idaho State Dental Association at 208-343-7543 or www.isdaweb.com.

- Illinois: The Illinois State Dental Society is online at www.isds.org, or call them at 217-525-1407. Programs include Donated Dental Services, 1-800-893-1685, and Take 2 Foster Care Referral at 1-888-286-2447.

- Indiana: The Indiana Dental Association at 317-634-2610 or www.indental.org offers a program called Give Kids a Smile to help children get the dental care they need.

- Iowa: Go to www.iowadental.org, or call 515-986-5606 to learn more about the Iowa Dental Association's new Iowa Missions of Mercy project, which will debut it 2008.

- Kansas: Call the Kansas Dental Association at 785-272-7360, or go to www.ksdentalfoundation.org to learn more about charitable dental care in your area.

- Kentucky: The Kentucky Dental Association has a Denture Access program designed to assist residents who are financially incapable of paying the total amount for a set of dentures.

To learn more about this and other programs, call 502-489-9121, or go to www.kyda.org.

For Your Health _____

Are you looking for a specific type of dental care but aren't sure if you can find it at a reasonable reduced cost in your state? Call your state dental association and tell them your situation and what you need. Just because your issue isn't on the website doesn't mean someone can't help you solve the problem once you're on the phone with them.

◆ Louisiana: Look under "Consumers and Community Service" for a long list of programs offered in the state. Go to www.222. ladental.org, or call 225-926-1986 to find out more.

◆ Maine: Call the Maine Dental Association at 207-622-7900, or go to www.medental.org to learn if there are programs in the state for the uninsured.

◆ Massachusetts: The Massachusetts Dental Society offers information on resources for uninsured residents if you click on "For the Public" at www.massdental.org, or call 508-480-9797.

◆ Michigan: Call the Michigan Dental Society at 517-372-9070, or go to www.smilemichigan.com to learn more about the community dental programs, which are listed by county.

◆ Minnesota: The Minnesota Dental Association at 612-767-8400 or www.mndental.org encourages dentists to offer care to low-income children through Give Kids a Smile.

◆ Mississippi: Call the Mississippi Dental Association at 601-982-0442, or go to www.msdental.org to learn more about public assistance programs.

◆ Missouri: Call the Missouri Dental Association at 573-634-3436, or go to www.resources.modental.org/pdf/Health/MISC/Low_Income_Clinics.pdf for a list of state providers.

◆ Montana: Call the Montana Dental Association at 406-443-2061, or go to www.mtdental.org to learn more about charitable care and the Give Kids a Smile program.

◆ Nebraska: The Nebraska Dental Association at 402-476-1704 and at www.nedental.org/Public/NMOM2007.htm explains the Mission of Mercy program for those who can't afford dental care.

◆ Nevada: Call the Nevada Dental Association at 702-255-4211, or go to www.nvda.org to learn more about care for uninsured residents.

◆ New Hampshire: Call the New Hampshire Dental Association at 603-225-5961, or go to www.nhds.org to learn more about care for uninsured residents.

◆ New Jersey: The New Jersey Dental Association website, www.njda.org, lists a number of programs for uninsured residents. Click on public and your oral health, or call 732-721-9400.

◆ New Mexico: Call the New Mexico Dental Association at 502-294-1368, or go to www.nmdental.org to learn more about care for uninsured residents.

◆ New York: Call the New York Sate Dental Association at 518-465-0044, or go to www.nysdental.org to find out more about care for uninsured residents.

◆ North Carolina: To learn more about the state health care endowment program for uninsured residents, go to www.ncdental.org/endowment.htm, the website for the North Carolina Website Society, or call 919-677-1396.

◆ Ohio: The Ohio Dental Association lists numerous programs for the uninsured on its website, www.oda.org/gendeninfo/programs.cfm, or call 614-486-2700.

◆ Oklahoma: Go to the Oklahoma Dental Association at www.okda.org, or call 405-848-8873 to find out about programs for uninsured residents.

◆ Oregon: Go to the Oregon Dental Association website, www.oregondental.org, and click on Community Programs, or call 503-218-2010 to learn more about dental care options.

◆ Pennsylvania: The Pennsylvania Dental Association website has a list of community clinics as well as senior citizen care resources on its website, www.padental.org, or call 717-234-5941.

◆ Rhode Island: Go to the Rhode Island Dental Association at www.ridental.org, or call 401-732-6833 to find out about programs for uninsured residents.

◆ South Carolina: The South Carolina Dental Association lists numerous free clinics around the state on its website, www.scda.org, or call 803-750-2277.

◆ South Dakota: Go to the South Dakota Dental Association at www.sddental.org, or call 605-224-9133 to find out about programs for uninsured residents.

◆ Tennessee: Go to the Tennessee Dental Association at www.tenndental.org, or call 615-628-0208 to find out about programs for uninsured residents.

◆ Texas: The Texas Dental Association website, www.tda.org, offers numerous programs for residents under TDA Smiles, or call 512-443-3675.

◆ Utah: To learn about how Utah helps its residents get dental care, go to www.health.utah.gov/oralhealth, or call 801-261-5315.

◆ Vermont: Go to the Vermont State Dental Association at www.vsdas.org, or call 802-864-0115 to find out about programs for uninsured residents.

◆ Virginia: Go to the Virginia Dental Association at www.vadental.org, or call 804-261-1610 to find out about programs for uninsured residents.

> **Bet You Didn't Know**
>
> You can always negotiate payment with a dentist just as you would any other doctor.

◆ Washington: Go to the Oral Health section of the Washington State Dental Association at www.wohfkidsconnect.com/home to learn more about programs for the uninsured. Or call 206-448-1914.

◆ West Virginia: Go to the West Virginia Dental Association at www.wvdental.org, or call 304-344-5246 to find out about programs for uninsured residents.

- ◆ Wisconsin: Look under Community Activities on the Wisconsin Dental Association website, www.wda.org, or call 414-276-4520 to learn more about programs.

- ◆ Wyoming: Go to the Wyoming Dental Association at www.wyda. org, or call 307-237-1186 to find out about programs for uninsured residents.

Remember the usefulness of a state's website may not indicate the state's actual ability to help its residents with dental care. Call the association to find out more about community programs.

Low-Cost Vision Care

According to the National Eye Institute, many state and national resources regularly provide aid to people with vision problems. The National Eye Institute, which supports eye research, does not help individuals pay for eye care. However, if you are in need of financial aid to assess or treat an eye problem, you might contact one or more of the following programs.

Organizations That Can Help

Organizations that offer help for uninsured people who need vision care include:

- ◆ EyeCare America, a public service foundation of the American Academy of Ophthalmology (AAO), provides comprehensive eye exams and care for up to one year, often at no out-of-pocket expense to eligible callers through its Senior and Diabetes EyeCare Programs. Its Glaucoma EyeCare Program provides a glaucoma eye exam. The EyeCare America Children's EyeCare Program educates parents and primary care providers about the importance of early childhood (newborn through 36 months of age) eye care. Call 1-800-222-EYES (3937), or go to www. eyecareamerica.org.

- ◆ Vision USA, run by the American Optometric Association (AOA), provides free eye care to uninsured, low-income workers and their families. Call 1-800-766-4466, or go to www.aoa.org/x5607.xml.

For Your Health

You can use prescription services for medications related to eye problems. Try the Medicine Program, which helps people enroll in the many patient assistance programs that provide prescription medicine free-of-charge to those in need. The program works in cooperation with the patient's doctor. Call 1-866-694-3893, or go to www.themedicineprogram.com. Or try the Partnership for Prescription Assistance, which offers a single point of access to more than 475 public and private patient assistance programs, including more than 150 programs offered by pharmaceutical companies. Call 1-888-477-2669, or go to www.pparx.org.

◆ The Lions Clubs International, a fraternal organization, provides financial assistance to individuals for eye care through its local clubs. Go to its website, www.LionsClub.org, and click on the club locator button. If you are unable to find your local Lions club, contact the LCIF Grant Programs Department at 630-571-5466 x393.

◆ Mission Cataract USA, a program coordinated by the Volunteer Eye Surgeons' Association, provides free cataract surgery to people of all ages who have no other means to pay. Surgeries are scheduled annually on one day, usually in May. Call 1-800-343-7265, or go to www.missioncataractUSA.org.

◆ The Knights Templar Eye Foundation provides assistance for eye surgery for people who are unable to pay or receive adequate assistance from current government agencies or similar sources. Call 847-490-3838, or go to www.knightstemplar.org/ktef.

◆ The National Keratoconus Assistance Foundation provides financial support to patients who need surgical and optometric treatment for keratoconus and other corneal problems. Go to www.nkcaf.org.

◆ InfantSEE is a public health program designed to ensure early detection of eye conditions in babies. Member optometrists provide a free comprehensive infant eye assessment to children younger than one year. Call 1-888-396-3937, or go to www.infantsee.org.

◆ Sight for Students is a Vision Service Plan (VSP) program that provides eye exams and glasses to children 18 years and younger whose families cannot afford vision care. Call 1-888-290-4964, or go to www.sightforstudents.org.

◆ New Eyes for the Needy provides vouchers for the purchase of new prescription eyeglasses. Call 973-376-4903, or go to www. neweyesfortheneedy.org.

Disease-Specific Eye Issues

Because patients with illnesses, such as diabetes, are at risk for eye problems, many health foundations offer tests and screening opportunities for those who suffer with long-term problems.

◆ If you have diabetes and qualify for Medicare or another public health insurance program, you may be able to get a dilated eye exam to check for diabetic eye disease. Your doctor will decide how often you need this exam.

◆ If you are at risk for glaucoma because of diabetes (even if there is a family history) or if you are an African American age 50 or older, some public health insurance programs will pay for an eye exam once a year. You may have to pay part of the cost. To find out more, call 1-800-633-4227.

If you have another illness, ask your doctor if you need regular eye exams and if she can recommend an eye doctor who provides this type of care to her patients. Some doctors will work together to help each other's patients.

Insurance for Your Eyes

Vision care is not just about the risk of blindness. Some people, of course, deal with poor eyesight, eye strain, and other eye issues for most of their lives. You may need vision insurance because of the cost of glasses or contacts rather than because you are worried about another type of eye health.

Vision insurance plans typically help defray costs of eye exams, eyewear, and other vision services and screenings.

Whether you want a comprehensive eye exam, eyeglasses, contact lenses, or laser eye surgery, you need to know that a vision plan typically doesn't cover 100 percent of your benefits, but, if you know you will have regular vision expenses, they can help reduce the expense.

Because vision insurance plans typically use networks of providers for services just like other health insurance plans, there are rarely managed care options for vision insurance. In fact, your best option may be to find a doctor that you like and trust and ask what insurance she takes. Then see if she can help you get a plan that works for both of you.

Benefits Packages and Discount Plans

Vision insurance typically comes in the form of either a vision benefits package or a discount vision plan. A typical vision benefits package provides eye care services in exchange for an annual premium or membership fee, a yearly deductible (a dollar amount) for each enrolled member, and a co-pay (a smaller dollar amount) each time a member accesses a service.

Meanwhile, a discount vision plan provides eye care at fixed discounted rates after an annual premium or membership fee and a deductible are paid.

> **Code Red**
>
> If you are interested in LASIK or PRK refractive surgery, remember these are usually considered elective surgical procedures, and it's possible your plan will not cover this surgery. Be sure to ask before you buy the insurance or schedule the appointment.

With a vision benefits package, you can expect to pay:

- ◆ A monthly premium or membership fee ranging from $0 to $12.
- ◆ A deductible of $0 to $35.
- ◆ A co-pay of $10 to $15 for each network service.
- ◆ Expenses for out-of-network services that go above and beyond plan allowances.

With a vision discount plan, you can expect to pay:

◆ A monthly premium or membership fee ranging from $0 to $12.

◆ A deductible of $0 to $35.

◆ A fixed discount price for each service you receive from a network provider or expenses for out-of-network services above and beyond plan allowances.

If you purchase an individual vision insurance plan, you will be billed monthly or annually.

Questions to Ask

Ask the vision insurance plan representative these questions:

◆ Does the plan allow out-of-network providers?

◆ Do out-of-network providers need to be approved by the vision insurance company in order for me to receive reimbursements?

◆ How do I request reimbursements for out-of-network services?

◆ What amounts can I expect to be reimbursed for each service?

For Your Health

Another option is to see an eye doctor and pay cash; then go online to order eyeglasses and contact lenses.

◆ How much is the deductible I must pay before the insurance company begins to pay its share of the expenses?

◆ How much is my co-pay for each service?

◆ Are there limits to what the plan will pay for any of the services?

Before you buy a Discount Vision Plan, ask:

◆ How much is the deductible I must pay before discounts apply?

◆ What discounted rate can I expect to pay out-of-pocket for each service?

◆ To whom do I pay the discount amounts? The vision insurance company? A primary care provider? Or each provider separately?

◆ How do I pay for services? Do I use a prepaid discount card, pre-paid coupons, cash, check, or credit card?

The Least You Need to Know

◆ Dental care is the type of medical attention that uninsured people want the most, but it is often the type of care even insured people don't get.

◆ Paying for teeth cleanings and check-ups will pay in the long run, since almost all expensive dental care can be discovered and helped earlier rather than later.

◆ Numerous organizations will help uninsured patients with vision care, especially if the problem has occurred in connection with other health conditions.

◆ You can negotiate on the cost of dental and vision care paid for in cash just as you can with other medical services.

◆ It pays to contact your state to learn more about dental and vision programs designed to help those without insurance.

Chapter 11

Elective Procedures and Surgery

In This Chapter

- ◆ Making a plan
- ◆ Negotiating the cost
- ◆ Who to hire
- ◆ Information you'll need
- ◆ Going out of the country

Think we're only talking about nose jobs when we politely write the words, Elective Surgery? *Au contraire.* For many people, with or without insurance, gallbladder removal, hysterectomies, hernia repairs and other procedures might all be considered elective because they can often be scheduled ahead of time at the patient's convenience.

If paying for the cost of these surgeries is all up to you (and might total in the tens of thousands), you have to make a decision about both your physical health and financial health.

A surgery is elective when you make a choice about whether or not and when to have it rather than having the choice made for you by an emergency, such as an accident or appendicitis.

The good news is that elective surgeries are actually easier to pay for with a well-thought-out plan. In fact, when surgery is elective, you can actually comparison shop for doctors, surgeons, hospitals, and all other services you'll need. And that means that, while overall your cost will no doubt be expensive, few surgeries are cheap, you can still save money and, perhaps best of all, pay for the whole thing over time rather than in one lump sum.

Making a Plan

Chances are, you went to your primary care physician and/or specialist who told you that you need a specific procedure to regain or maintain your good health. Any patient, even one with great insurance, should consider getting a second opinion even if this means an extra cost of a few hundred dollars because you are paying for the doctor's visit out-of-pocket. You may save money in the long run, especially if it turns out you don't need a procedure or you could have an alternate procedure in its place.

Code Red

The doctor who gives you a diagnosis does not have to be and often won't be the surgeon who operates on you. You should shop for a surgeon just as you, we hope, shopped for a specialist to help you with your case.

Once you have made a decision about the procedure you are going to have, you need to create a two-part plan that includes your physical plan and your financial plan.

The physical plan involves any presurgical steps you need to take, such as tests and procedures, any items you might need (slippers and robe for the hospital, for example), as well as expenses you can expect during your surgery and hospital stay. Also figure out what you'll need after your surgery. Will you need help caring for yourself? Will you need a wheelchair? A bedpan? A hospital bed?

You also need to find a doctor and, possibly, an anesthesiologist. While it's certainly true that the hospital will provide many of these specialists, it's also true that these experts will be sending you a bill. Since you can pick some of the specialists who will take care of you, you can also use this time to work out discounts or payment plans with them. In fact, their prices and willingness to work with you on payment may play into your decision-making process.

Choosing a Hospital

This worksheet, published by the Department of Health and Human Services, gives you some questions to ask when you are choosing a hospital. You want to find the answers to these questions because research has shown that some hospitals simply do a better job with specific surgeries. For example, hospitals that do a greater number of the same surgeries, such as valve replacements or hysterectomies, have better outcomes for their patients.

Look for a hospital that:

◆ Is accredited by the Joint Commission on Accreditation of Healthcare Organizations.

◆ Is rated highly by state or consumer or other groups.

◆ Is one where your doctor has privileges and typically works. If not, you will most likely be under the care of another doctor while at the hospital.

◆ Has experience with your condition. For example, general hospitals handle a wide range of routine conditions, such as hernias and pneumonia. Specialty hospitals have extensive experience with specific conditions, such as cancer, or certain populations, such as children or women.

◆ Has had success with your condition. Research shows that hospitals that do many of the same types of procedures tend to have better success with them. Ask your doctor or the hospital how often the procedure is done there, how often the doctor does the procedure, and what are the patient outcomes.

◆ Monitors surgical outcomes and works to improve its own quality of care.

◆ Meets national quality standards. Hospitals can choose to be surveyed by the Joint Commission on Accreditation of Healthcare Organizations (JCAHO) to make sure they meet certain quality standards. The standards address the quality of staff and equipment, and—most recently—the hospital's success in treating and curing patients. If a hospital meets those standards, it becomes accredited (gets a seal of approval). Reviews are done at least every three years, and most hospitals participate in this program.

You can call 630-792-5800 to order JCAHO performance reports. It's free. Or go to the JCAHO web site at www.jcaho.org for a hospital's performance report or for its accreditation status.

Of course, typically, most of these checklists also suggest that you find a hospital that is part of your health insurance plan, but if that doesn't apply to you, we suggest you choose a hospital that will work with you before and after the procedure to ease any financial stress.

Bet You Didn't Know

All Canadians receive comprehensive, universal, portable, and accessible health insurance. Primary care physicians, who are typically fee-for-service, submitting claims to the health plan, account for 51 percent of Canada doctors, providing care and overseeing specialists, hospitals, tests, and prescription drugs. Over 95 percent of hospitals in Canada are private nonprofits, and taxes finance the whole system. Canadians do not pay deductibles or co-payments, although most elective surgery isn't covered. Two thirds of Canadians said their families had to wait longer for medical service in the last year than they thought was reasonable, mostly because there are 2.1 doctors per 1,000 persons, 25 percent lower than the average in other leading industrialized countries. In fact, some provinces work with U.S. doctors for quicker service.

Most states and some medical consumer groups create reports that rank hospitals. Besides helping consumers make informed choices, these also encourage hospitals to improve their quality of care. For example, businesses, doctors, and hospitals make up the Cleveland Health Quality Choice Program.

Coding Specifics

Medical providers use a standardized system of numbers or codes for all services. Government programs, such as Medicare and Medicaid, require these codes, which now have become the norm for the entire medical and health insurance industries. Each code specifies a specific procedure or service, and each of those services has a related cost or charge. In other words, when a code is entered into the system, a doctor, hospital, lab, or other provider will receive a reimbursement based on that set of numbers.

These standards are understood by health professionals who have guides to the codes, but they are problematic for two reasons. First, no one else understands what each code means. Second, hospitals and other providers can potentially *upcode* services as a way to charge more.

def•i•ni•tion

Upcoding is when medical providers list a code on a claim representing a service or procedure that was more expensive than the one that was actually provided.

Because Medicare, Medicaid, and other health insurers may have agreed-upon prices for every procedure, providers can't charge any amount they want to for a specific service or procedure. So medical providers may be tempted to use the wrong codes in order to make more money.

Since all you can see on the claim form is strings of numbers that represent codes for what was done, it can be challenging to determine what you are actually being charged for.

Insurance companies employ claims examiners to determine the validity and accuracy of medical claims. As an individual without insurance, you are the person most at risk to be overcharged due to inaccurate coding and billing. After all, you don't have the expertise of an insurance company behind you.

You may not have the knowledge to understand every code and therefore, every charge associated with each code. But, you do have the ability to question the codes and charges. You have the right to an explanation in simple language to every charge on the bill. Simply call the billing department and ask.

More to the point, while you are shopping for a hospital, you can discuss the cost of the operation up front and negotiate a global fee, eliminating the need to "decode" all those numbers. At the same time be sure to ask whether you will be billed separately by your doctors and if you (or the hospital) can negotiate rates with them as well. It is possible that you may receive separate bills for service from the surgeon, anesthesiologist, pathologist, and any number of consultants who may be involved with the case. It is often easier to negotiate on fees ahead of time when you still have the option of going elsewhere for elective surgery.

Negotiating the Cost

The most important thing to remember before you start to negotiate the cost of your procedure is that the more research you do before you start to talk to the hospital or other provider, the more likely you will be able to agree on a reasonable price. In this case, knowledge really is power.

For example, you will get a more reasonable price on your procedure if you remember that hospitals charge uninsured patients full price while insured patients usually have prenegotiated discounts. So talk to the finance department about the price an insurance company would pay for the same surgery.

Likewise, you will be empowered if you remember that Medicaid pays lower prices than even private insurance companies, so ask what Medicaid considers reasonable reimbursement for the procedure.

Finally, you have power if you remember that many hospitals can be reimbursed for charity care they provide. In other words, if the hospital claims that they can't do your procedure for free, explain to them that you know they can get some credit for charity care. In this case be prepared to prove you qualify by producing financial records. With all this in mind, you can begin to negotiate the cost of your procedure:

1. First, explain to your doctor that you don't have insurance and you're going to try to negotiate payment with the hospital. If he's on your side, he may be able to help.

2. Talk to your doctor and anyone else involved in the procedure, such as an anesthesiologist, to find out exactly what they expect to do. Get a detailed list of each step and the people and expenses involved.

3. Call the hospital, and find someone in the billing department who you can always be in contact with. By developing a relationship with one individual, you won't have to talk with different people, repeating your story each time you speak.

For Your Health

Shopping for a hospital is different from comparison shopping for other big-ticket items. You need to think about the money you're going to spend, but you also need to think about your health and your well-being. The comfort you feel with a particular doctor as well as in a particular hospital matters. Likewise, don't forget about proximity. Spending a little extra money may be worth while if you are closer to home and more people can visit you.

4. Explain your situation openly and honestly. Explain, too, that you are shopping around to find a hospital that will work with you on the bill. Get the prices for individual items, such as the room rate, medications, and any professional services.

5. It's very possible that the first person you speak with won't be the one who can make decisions, so write down each person's name and all the information he gives you.

6. Do more research. Go home with the prices they've offered, and call around. Find out if other hospitals have vastly different prices. Check to see how these prices compare with those offered to insurance companies.

7. Return to the last person you spoke with—hopefully, someone who can make pricing decisions—and make them an offer.

8. The billing department might possibly suggest you take out a loan. Typically they ask to be paid in advance, by credit card, or within 30 days for a cash transaction. It's possible they may allow you to set up a payment plan. It doesn't hurt to ask.

In other words, do your best to work with the hospital and other providers to both pay the bill and reduce the price so that it is fair to both of you. This is what an insurance company would do and, at this point, you are your best advocate. The hospital and providers need to be paid as much as you need health care.

Hiring Private Nurses

While you're looking for a doctor and hospital, you might also consider trying to find a nurse to help you when you arrive home. Many *private-duty nurses* now work in a home or a hospital to not only care for the patient but also to advocate for him if he needs help in the hospital or with the system.

def•i•ni•tion

Private Duty Nursing (PDN) is defined as the provision of medically necessary, complex, skilled nursing care in the home by a registered nurse (RN) or a licensed practical nurse (LPN). The purpose of private duty nursing is to assess, monitor, and provide skilled nursing care in the home on an hourly basis; to assist in the transition of care from a more acute setting to home; and to teach competent caregivers the assumption of this care when the condition of the member is stabilized.

A private duty nurse can earn anywhere from $20 to $100 an hour depending on the location and their specialization and licensing. Sometimes PDNs provide only medical care while others do more personal care, such as helping someone in the bathroom and with grooming.

If you don't want or need a private nurse but do want someone to help you out at home or in the hospital, consider paying a friend or relative (if she can't do it for free, of course) to help you out. Many people without insurance are afraid they won't get the care they need, especially if they are undergoing a serious operation. Having an advocate will help you feel more secure and give you better care, should you need it.

To find a private nurse, call a certified home health agency or local social services office as well as nursing agencies.

Information You Need on Hand at All Times

During your phone calls, while you're at the doctor, and when you're in the hospital, always have copies of your medical and financial records with you. Don't bring originals with you, and always be sure the providers take copies—not yours—for their own records.

Likewise, make notes about who you speak with and when so that all of your information is accurate. This will reduce the potential run-around you will get from providers.

For Your Health

> I know a patient who was uninsured and needed elective eye surgery. He had the resources to pay cash, but the "list price" of the surgery was very expensive. By negotiating in advance with the hospital and the ophthalmologist, he was able to save nearly 50 percent on the cost of the procedure.

Going Overseas for Medical Treatment

So after all the negotiating and comparison shopping, perhaps you are still left with the knowledge that whatever procedure you need (or want) is just too expensive for you. Do you have another alterative?

These days, more and more Americans are traveling overseas or sometimes just across the border to get less expensive medical care. Of course, not everyone thinks this is a good idea. Price isn't the only consideration when you're having a medical procedure. But for many Americans, the promise of lower-cost surgeries, coupled with the good reputation of the medical systems in some other countries, add up to a better option than the American health-care system.

This option has been especially true for cosmetic surgery, which most health insurance companies don't cover anyway, so even insured Americans have to pay these expenses out of their own pocket.

> **Bet You Didn't Know**
>
> If the surgery you want is cosmetic, many overseas hospitals and clinics offer packages for multiple procedures and sometimes even include spa services.

Comparison Shopping

Of course, if you go overseas you have to do some—if not more—comparison shopping. It's not as if other countries have health systems that cover Americans. On the other hand, overseas surgeries is a competitive market. In clinics throughout the world, the cost may be half to one-third of what the same surgery would cost in the United States. And because these clinics and hospitals want to appeal to Americans, the cost sometimes includes hotel stays and meals.

You'll need to include the following expenses when you comparison shop for an overseas procedure: air travel, hotel accommodations, travel to the hospital from the hotel, meals, nurses (if necessary), medications, and costs of supplies your clinic doesn't cover, which might mean bandages and dressings. Remember, American hospitals charge for these items, so you'll want to find out if your overseas hospital does, too.

You must also consider another added expense, which can be a big one. You can't necessarily fly home the day after having major surgery. In fact, most overseas hospitals insist on at least ten days of post-surgery recovery period and some, two weeks. That's why spa services are offered at some clinics; it's supposed to be like a vacation!

These days, Americans are traveling abroad not only for cosmetic surgery but also for hip replacements and even heart surgery. One hospital in India, Bumrungrad, had 55,000 foreign patients in 2006, and three-quarters of them came from the United States, almost all of them for noncosmetic procedures.

Bet You Didn't Know

France covers all workers of legal residence, as well as the spouses and children of those workers, with a national health insurance plan. Many people also buy additional insurance to complement or supplement the state-run program. Patients do not need a referral to see a specialist. There are two types of hospitals in France with varying types of reimbursements. A 1999 poll found that 78.2 percent of French citizens were very or fairly satisfied with their health-care system, while 21.1 percent were dissatisfied.

Even though you are traveling out of the country for the procedure, you'll need to get many of your preliminary exams, such as lab tests and some X-rays, in the United States. In fact, many of the foreign hospitals will only accept you as a patient once they have deemed you a good candidate for surgery.

Of course, if you have dual citizenship or are a foreign national, maybe you can go home to your country of origin for health care.

Bet You Didn't Know

Most Germans receive health-care coverage through the state health insurance plans. Employers and employees each pay half of the contributions. Additional subsidies for coverage are offered for the poor, the unemployed, and the elderly. Less than 0.2 percent of the population is uninsured.

Since 2004, in a deeply unpopular reform, Germans have had to pay 10 euros per quarter to see a general practitioner. Members of the health-care plan must contribute toward the cost of prescription drugs, wound dressings and bandages; and 15 or 20 percent of the cost of other items. Long waits are a particular problem; 19.4 percent of Germans report waiting more than 12 weeks between seeing a specialist and receiving surgery.

Issues to Consider

Some of the more superficial issues that arise when considering overseas medical procedures include not liking the food in a foreign country, feeling isolated and far from home, and not speaking the language of the other patients.

Most important, of course, you need to consider the matter of safety. Insurance or not, you will not be as legally protected in terms of patient's rights and citizen's rights in another country. Do your research to be sure you are in good hands. How good is the doctor and the hospital?

What if something goes wrong? What if you can't fend for yourself? Will someone be with you to help out?

Some of the countries that encourage American patients include Brazil, Canada, Mexico, Thailand, India, and the nations in the European Union.

Bet You Didn't Know

The United Kingdom's National Health Service delegates most patient care to local Primary Care Trusts (PCTs). Some UK residents opt for private insurance rather than coverage under the NHS. Visits to primary care physicians, specialists, and in-patient care and tests are free. Other services, such as prescriptions, dental care, and vision care are dependent on circumstances—sometimes individuals pay; sometimes it is subsidized. 41.2 percent of Britons report waiting more than 12 weeks between getting a diagnosis and having surgery. And local finances matter—some PCTs lack doctors and nurses.

It is important to repeat that spending more on health care does not necessarily mean you will get better care, according to Harvard Medical School (2007) and other researchers. No correlation exists between the price of health care and its quality.

Bet You Didn't Know

Japan's universal health coverage offers National Health Insurance and Employees' Health Insurance. Premiums are about 4 percent of a monthly salary; the employer pays half and the employee half. Those covered under Employee Health Insurance pay 20 percent of their medical costs when hospitalized and 30 percent of the costs for out-patient care, as well as for prescription drugs. Conditions not covered include orthodontic work, cosmetic surgery, vaccinations, abortions, injuries incurred while drunk or fighting, and treatment outside of Japan. The Japanese population is getting older, and younger working citizens will be outnumbered by elderly, which will stress the system. In Japan, hospital stays are two to three times longer than in the West.

Ask Around

As with any type of comparison shopping, the best way to find what you need is to ask around. Don't be shy about telling friends, co-workers, and even your doctor that you are considering going out of the country for the health care you need. As these options become more common, more likely others will know of people who have done this. Asking for information as well as recommendations can only help you.

No federal agency or organization oversees or assists Americans who go out of the country specifically for medical care, so, at this point, there are no official recommendations or guidelines to help you make this choice.

The Least You Need to Know

◆ If it's not an emergency, you always have the option to comparison shop when it comes to health care. Call around to hospitals, and doctors, to see what they charge for the supplies you need.

◆ Consider hiring a private nurse, who can also act as an advocate, to be sure you get the physical care you need as well as the emotional support you want.

◆ When you speak to a provider, have all your medical and financial information nearby, as well as a notebook to keep track of what you are told.

◆ Care is not free for those who live in other countries, and it won't be free for you if you go out of the country for medical treatment. Aside from the medical expenses, you also must deal with hotel stays, food, and travel expenses. Do not consider going out of the country without researching safety and comparing the prices to local costs.

Part 3

When You Need Care Now

According to government statistics, more than 300,000 Americans go to the emergency room every day. But that doesn't mean there are 300,000 healthcare emergencies. Knowing when to use the emergency room, and when not to, is an important aspect of health care for everyone, especially the uninsured. In this part we also provide strategies for dealing with denied claims and paying the bill on your own time. You have more negotiating power than you think.

Chapter 12

When to Use—and Avoid—the Emergency Room

In This Chapter

- ◆ Use the emergency room judiciously
- ◆ The emergency room is not free for anyone
- ◆ Symptoms for emergency room use
- ◆ Dealing with the bills

According to government statistics, more than 300,000 Americans go to the emergency room every day. And everyone is scared and worried when he goes to an emergency room, but for someone without insurance, the trip is often taken too late and with the extra fear of how he will pay the bill.

Why is the trip taken too late? Because when someone is worried about how he is going to pay a bill, he puts off going to the doctor or emergency room so he won't have another bill to deal with. Unfortunately, this kind of wait-and-see game can be dangerous and end with a patient needing more expensive care due to the increased severity of the illness or problem.

Of course, that doesn't mean every sick person should go straight to an emergency room. In fact, whether or not someone has insurance shouldn't determine when he goes to the emergency room. One criteria alone should determine emergency room visits: if the health event is an emergency.

Defining an Emergency

When is a medical condition an emergency? According to The American College of Emergency Physicians (ACEP) these warning signs indicate a medical emergency:

♦ Difficulty breathing, shortness of breath

♦ Chest or upper abdominal pain or pressure

♦ Fainting, sudden dizziness, weakness

♦ Changes in vision

♦ Confusion or changes in mental status

♦ Any sudden or severe pain

♦ Uncontrolled bleeding

♦ Severe or persistent vomiting or diarrhea

♦ Coughing or vomiting blood

♦ Suicidal feelings

♦ Difficulty speaking

♦ Unusual abdominal pain

> **Code Red**
>
> Children have unique medical problems and may display different symptoms than adults. Symptoms that are serious for a child may not be as serious for an adult. Children may also be unable to communicate their condition, which means an adult will have to interpret the behavior. Always get immediate medical attention if you think your child is having a medical emergency.

You or your loved one needs to use your instincts when it comes to making the decision about an emergency. If you think the medical condition is life-threatening or the person's condition will worsen on the way to the hospital, then you need to call 9-1-1 and have your local emergency medical services provider come to you.

Really, when you are sick or hurt, whether or not you have insurance should not be the key issue. The key issue is whether to go to the emergency room or not based on your symptoms. Most of your decision will boil down to common sense, and you have to understand that you can't know what your diagnosis will be ahead of time, and sometimes people choose to go to the emergency room when they don't need to. No one has perfect knowledge.

Calling 9-1-1

Not too many years ago, people had to find the right phone number in an emergency. If there was a fire, people phoned the fire department. If there was a crime, they called the police. If someone got hurt, they had to call an ambulance. Finding a number for any of these emergency workers could be very confusing, especially if a person was in a hurry or in an unfamiliar area.

Today, it's as simple as dialing 911. With those three numbers, you can reach the fire department, the police, or an ambulance. When you call 911, an emergency operator, called a dispatcher, immediately connects you to the person you need. But, here's the thing—what happens next— let's say an ambulance arrives—may cost you.

Let's suppose, for an example, that your car is rear-ended. Someone who saw the accident calls the ambulance, which quickly shows up. The emergency medical technician (EMT) asks you how you feel, and you say your neck hurts. The next thing you know they have strapped you to the board, and the siren is screaming. You're headed for the emergency room.

> **Bet You Didn't Know**
>
> Chances are you probably have car insurance even if you don't have health insurance. If you're in an accident and are conscious, call your car insurance agent first. If you think you need to see a doctor, ask if your coverage includes any kind of medical treatment.

Of course, if you're hurt, go to the hospital. Don't worry about the bill ahead of getting treatment if you need it. Before you let the ambulance driver take you anywhere, though, you need to know two things. First, you don't have to go with them if you don't think you need to, and second, that ride is not free.

Depending on who provides the ambulance service , you're probably going to get a bill. The municipality in which you've had your accident might run the ambulance. If you have no insurance, what happens to the bill will depend on the town's policy toward the uninsured. They may have an internal policy saying that if you're a resident of the town, they won't send you a bill. But, they may send you a bill regardless of where you live.

The town may or may not insist you pay the bill once you tell them you have no insurance. They may just write it off, but you should always call them and tell them your situation as well as thank them for the service they provided.

These days, however, private companies run many ambulance services, and they will absolutely bill you no matter where you live. They might also be more insistent that you get into the ambulance whether you need it or not. Once again, though, don't ignore the bill. Instead, call them and ask what you're being billed for. Figure out what they are asking you to pay and ask some questions. Was the trip to the hospital 16 miles? Did you really get oxygen? Did you need those things? Remember, you have the right to refuse the ambulance if you feel you are not injured (this assumes you are not legally intoxicated or suicidal).

> **Bet You Didn't Know**
>
> You are actually in the perfect negotiating situation when you get billed after the medical services have happened. They can't refuse you service because it's already been provided, and before you pay you have a chance to negotiate the fee or a payment plan.

Tell the ambulance service that you have no insurance and that you want to work with them but that you don't have the money to simply pay the bill. Once you've agreed on a reasonable fee or charge, then work out a payment plan if necessary.

Do You Need to Go to the Hospital?

One thing you can do before heading to the emergency room is call the hospital and see if they have an outpatient service or a Dial-A-Nurse option. Some nurse hot-lines are subscription services. Doctors join them so when someone calls with a problem, the service will recommend that person to the doctor who subscribes. You can use these services for minor emergencies, as well as for everyday illness, to get advice and recommendations.

To test this type of service, we had Paula, the mom of an eight-month-old, call a local 800 ask-a-nurse number when her baby was sick. Paula told the nurse that the baby had a fever but no other symptoms and the fever was low, 101.2. The nurse advised Paula (appropriately, according to her physician) to go to the pharmacy and buy some Tylenol, instead of going to the ER or even the pediatrician. Nevertheless, the nurse sounded a little nervous, and Paula's physician said that the usefulness of these services really depends on the caller giving thoughtful information as well as the nurse knowing what questions to ask to be sure that the advice she gives is appropriate. The nurse did offer to provide Paula with the name and contact information of a local doctor, but she didn't push Paula to make an unnecessary appointment.

Telephone *triage* is potentially difficult and risky. The nurse depends on the patient, or in this case his parent, to provide her with an accurate patient history and description of the symptoms, while the patient depends on the nurse to make the right diagnosis just on the basis of a phone call.

The other issue is that, depending on who runs the "free" service, the nurse may have a hidden agenda. In the case of a hotline run by the hospital or doctor, the nurse wants to find a good reason to advise you to go to the hospital, clinic, or one of their local doctors. In the case of the paid (usually by an insurer) service, the nurse is instructed to try to avoid having you come

> ### def•i•ni•tion
> **Triage** is the process of prioritizing sick or injured people for treatment according to the seriousness of the condition or injury. If you remember the TV show *M*A*S*H*, you know that hospital personnel triage emergency patients and decide who needs to go into the ER first.

to the doctor unnecessarily and instead route you to the most "cost effective" provider, such as buying a painkiller at the drugstore. It's important for you, the patient, to be aware that a subtle bias may be at work here.

At the Emergency Room

According to federal law, the Emergency Treatment and Active Labor Act (EMTALA), a hospital emergency department has to provide all comers regardless of insurance status an appropriate screening exam and emergency care. Once the patient has been examined, if no emergency condition is present (as determined by the physician) the hospital is within its legal rights to discharge the patient without treatment, for example, an indigent patient who comes to the ER for chronic arthritis). However, by the time the screening exam is completed, most physicians believe they may as well (and ethically should) treat the patient anyway since they've already done the hard part (made the diagnosis).

> **For Your Health** _____
>
> If you can, bring a list of medications and allergies to the emergency room. Know the name of the medication you are taking, how often you take it, and for how long. A list of any medication allergies is important. Be sure to include medications, foods, insects, or any other product that may cause an allergic reaction. Also, bring a medical history form with you. ACEP has medical history forms available on its website.

Here are some realities:

◆ Most emergency physicians don't even know whether or not you have insurance unless they have a particular interest and take the time to look through the chart for the insurance information. So they pretty much treat everyone the same. Being polite and thoughtful will usually elicit a better response from providers than having good insurance.

◆ Nevertheless, the insurance issue does come up when a patient needs to be admitted or referred for follow-up. This varies by hospital, state, and locale, so it's hard to generalize. Usually the on-call specialist is obligated to see the emergency room patient at least once in follow-up.

Sometimes, the referral doctor may ask the emergency physician about the patient's insurance status. Very often, the physicians just say they don't know the insurance status, since they often don't. If the office staff screens uninsured patients out it may be helpful to remind them you were referred from the emergency room on their doctor's on call coverage day. They (probably) have an obligation to see you (at least once).

◆ Specialists on call may be less likely to come and see a patient in the ER if the patient isn't insured, but this often depends more on the time of day or night they are being called and what they are doing at the time. No surgeon who is scheduled in the OR at 7 A.M. is excited about coming to see anyone late at night, regardless of insurance status.

Many hospitals now have case managers who check on insurance status and utilization criteria used by insurance companies. These case managers sometimes try to persuade the doctor not to admit the patient if they don't think the bill will be paid. Or alternatively they may ask for a different diagnosis or documentation so that the (insured) patient will meet criteria.

For Your Health

Mental health patients and alcohol or drug detox patients may be offered admission (or not) based directly on their insurance status (depending on their diagnosis and the severity of illness).

Remember no patient who is acutely and seriously ill is turned away. This is pretty much true everywhere in the United States. Be aware, however, that the emergency physician's definition of acutely and seriously ill (the patient is at high risk of death or permanent disability) may be different from your own.

What About the Emergency Room Bill?

An emergency room visit has no average cost since so many factors come into play (location, type of hospital, problem you are seen for, length of stay, tests, etc.). But, no matter why you go to the emergency room, you will get a bill.

If you can, talk to the hospital's finance department to get a sense of the amount of the bill and their payment arrangements. The more upfront you can be about the cost of the bill and your situation, the more likely the hospital will be to work with you.

Hospitals are much more willing to make a financial plan with you than you might realize since billing and bill collection is a high expense (see Chapter 14).

Code Red

People like to talk about the health care safety net, which is supposed to catch all the people who "fall through the cracks" of the traditional health-care system. The "safety net" is to some degree a figment of the imagination employed to explain away the failings and lack of a coordinated system. The safety net should not be the emergency room, which is not designed to efficiently deal with all medical problems.

The Least You Need to Know

◆ If you are in a true emergency—a life-threatening condition—the hospital, by law, must see and care for you.

◆ For treatment of a chronic illness or for symptoms of a minor or nonemergency (such as a cold or flu), call the hospital to see if they have an outpatient clinic, which may be less expensive and more convenient than an emergency room visit.

◆ Call a hotline for advice if you aren't sure you need to see a doctor. If you can safely drive to the hospital rather than calling an ambulance, do so, as you will be billed for ambulance services.

◆ Work with the provider as soon as possible to get a handle on the cost of your bill and to work out a payment plan.

Chapter 13

The Denied Claim

In This Chapter

- ◆ Think like an insurance company
- ◆ Follow the rules and regulations
- ◆ Check out the appeals process
- ◆ Consider the need for a lawyer

So you think you've picked out a good insurance policy, or maybe you use government-subsidized insurance and feel you're safely covered. Then, you are in a car accident. It's not serious, but you do spend a night in the hospital while the doctors make sure you have no internal injuries. You hand over your insurance card, sign all the paperwork, and go home, relieved and happy that you are safe, and happy, too, that you have been good about paying your insurance.

Then, three weeks later, you get a two-page form with lots of numbers and codes on it. At the very bottom of the second page, you read: "Amount You Owe Provider—$9,300."

What?! As you look at the columns above that number, you see the word "denied" over and over again, as well as more numbers, all of which are less than the amount you were billed. For example:

Service Information	Service Date	Amount Billed	Not Covered	Covered
Spec Med Vis	12-15-07	563.00	563.00	0.00
Diag Med Ex	12-15-07	398.00	398.00	0.00

Now what do you do?

Why Health Insurance Doesn't Cover Everything

Before we get into the specifics of your situation in a profit-driven system, we think it would empower you to understand that system's intentions and way of doing business. If you understand the system, you can use the knowledge to your advantage.

The Concept of Moral Hazard

The American health insurance industry is built on the concept of moral hazard. This, in layperson terms, means that if the insurance company gives you, the consumer, the option of getting all the health care you need or want, they think you'll be greedy and pretend to be sick most of the time. So the insurance company, in its attempt to protect you from your own presumably greedy self, has decided to deny you coverage for some of the care you need. This way, the thinking goes, you won't overuse the system in an attempt to rip it off.

This theory of moral hazard explains why you are responsible for a co-pay to your doctor (if it were completely free, wouldn't you go all the time?), and why you have a deductible (if you didn't have to pay for health care, wouldn't you be sick more often?).

But, of course, we know this isn't really true.

The reality is that most of us don't want to be sick; nor do most of us want to go to the doctor, have surgery, or go to the dentist. Life is far better for the healthier and insured than for the sick and uninsured.

Bet You Didn't Know
The federal government has long struggled with the idea of a national single-payer health plan. And George W. Bush actually summed up the struggle succinctly in 2007: "The fundamental question is, what should we do about [health-care costs]? On that question, our nation has a clear choice. One option is to put more power in the hands of government by expanding federal health care programs and empowering bureaucrats to make medical decisions. The other option is to put more power in the hands of individuals, by making private health insurance more affordable and accessible and empowering people and their doctors to make the decisions that are right for them. That's the divide."

One problem with the moral hazard theory on which our nation's health care rests is that it also works in reverse. That is, it discourages people from using the health-care system even when it's necessary. The more money people are asked to pay for their care, the less they see the doctor. Then, when they are really sick, the more money it costs to treat them. In fact, it pays to get preventative care, but that's just what people cut down on when they don't have insurance.

And of course, another problem is that the moral hazard insurance system only applies to those who have limited amounts of money. If someone has plenty of money, he goes to see the doctor whenever he needs to, whether or not he is really sick, because money is no object.

Code Red

Some of the most frequently denied claims include inpatient hospital stays, psychiatric services, and other medical care made on behalf of adults who want services for children or elderly people.

Other Issues

So remember, the system is built to force you to pay for and justify the services you use. And keep in mind three more things when you deal with the insurance company, as well as the provider.

◆ First, not everyone is charged the same amount for a service. Providers charge different amounts for services depending on the deal your insurance company has with the provider as well as the specifics of your insurance policy.

◆ Second, hospitals and other providers sometimes "upcode" (see Chapter 11) as a way to charge more for services. So if you went to the hospital because of a car accident, was it really necessary that you stay overnight if you had no symptoms? Who made that decision? What tests were performed and why?

◆ Third, some tests and hospital stays may be ordered more to protect the doctor from being sued for a missed diagnosis than for any really significant risk.

Never be afraid to ask the doctor whether a test or procedure is really necessary, what the alternatives are, or how much it will cost. As a competent adult you always have the right to refuse treatment at any time or to sign out of the hospital. You may be asked to sign a waiver of liability (AMA—against medical advice), but you cannot be held or treated against your will. The only exception to this is if you are in some way mentally impaired or judged suicidal.

Much of the language in an insurance plan is vague at best. So, if your policy says it will pay for "medically necessary" treatment, who decides what is medically necessary? If the doctor at the hospital said it was medically necessary for you to be observed but the doctor (or a clerk) at the insurance company said it wasn't, who is the expert?

Some of the argument over your hospital bill is not between you and the provider but between the provider and the insurance company. However, you might still be getting bills and perhaps even phone calls because the hospital or other provider may take the chance that you'll simply pay the bill. Call the provider, and

> **Code Red**
>
> Even if your health insurance or health care is subsidized by a state health insurance policy or some form of Medicaid, you are not automatically covered for every procedure and service. You will still need to know how to deal with the various providers and insurers in order to protect your rights.

explain that your insurance company is disputing the charges and that you will not pay while that is happening.

How to Appeal a Denied Claim

No matter what kind of insurance you have, whether your plan is part of a group, employer-sponsored insurance, or government subsidized insurance, you will need to follow the exact process of filing an appeal because denial of coverage varies from plan to plan.

First, call the insurer to have someone explain what each charge is for and why they are denying coverage. Of course, take notes during each phone call related to your *claim*, and write down the names of people you spoke with, the date, and the information they gave you.

Follow up each call with a letter summarizing the conversation. Send the letter to your doctor or other provider and the insurance company. Always date the letter, and include the names and contact information of each person involved.

def•i•ni•tion

A **claim** is an official request for money or other benefits from an insurance company.

Likewise, keep copies of all records, including every notice and piece of correspondence, whether by e-mail or letter.

Also look into your specific state law that protects you if your claim is denied. Your insurance type and state of residence determine your specific safeguards, so we've included resources to help you get information tailored for your situation.

Once you understand which claims are being denied, ask your insurer to justify its decision in writing. Ask about the medical background of the person who made the denial decision. Also, ask the insurance company if it has an appeals form and process already laid out. Be sure you do this because if you don't follow the insurance company's rules, you may end up repeating all of these steps.

Once you get this information in the mail, call the provider (typically a hospital and doctor) and ask them to explain why those specific procedures or tests were done and why they feel they were necessary. Ask the

For Your Health

Your state insurance department is the best source of information on your legal rights. To find out more about your state's laws, contact NAIC Executive Headquarters, 2301 McGee Street, Suite 800, Kansas City, MO 64108-2662; phone 816-842-3600; or go to www.naic. org/state_web_map.htm.

provider to put that information in writing, and send that explanation to the insurance company.

If the insurer doesn't send adequate or appropriate justification for its decision, then explain that you believe the decision may be invalid and that you plan to take the decision to the state insurance board if you can't resolve the issue between yourselves.

Once you've heard from the provider about the treatments and their medical necessity, write back to the insurance company with the back-up from the provider. Explain why you think the denial decision should be overturned.

Be sure to use and include all of this information regardless of whether the insurance company's appeal form asks for it.

Bet You Didn't Know

If you have employer-provided insurance or insurance through COBRA, you're probably covered by the federal Employee Retirement Income Security Act (ERISA). This law sets legal guidelines for private employee benefit plans. ERISA mandates that your insurer must:

◆ Inform you about your plan's provisions, including how to file a claim

◆ Maintain an impartial process for reviewing appeals

◆ Meet certain deadlines in returning decisions on claims and appeals

◆ Speed up the process if your doctor declares your claim urgent

◆ Give you at least 180 days to file an appeal

If your insurance company isn't satisfying your requests, you still have some options.

If you have employer-sponsored insurance or group insurance through an organization, ask someone in the benefits department to support your appeal. This will add the weight of the whole organization to your complaint.

For Your Health

To learn even more about your rights, get a copy of "A Consumer Guide to Handling Disputes with Your Employer or Private Health Plan" sponsored by the Kaiser Family Foundation. This pamphlet helps consumers navigate their employer or private health plan's internal grievance procedure and external review programs of specific states. Go to www.kff.org/consumerguide/states.cfm to learn more.

It is most important that you file your appeal—as well as all of the supporting paperwork—on time. Most insurance companies stick to strict deadlines, such as 30, 60, or 90 days, in order to restrict your ability to fight for your rights. Do not try to fight these deadlines because that's a losing battle. Instead, follow those rules while you're trying to protect your financial rights.

Always be polite, respectful, and courteous during all these negotiations. Don't waste your time arguing over items that are clearly your responsibility to pay, especially if you have a deductible or a co-pay. Likewise, remember that your insurer (like you) would rather come to a friendly agreement than begin a potentially expensive process to resolve your appeal.

Bet You Didn't Know

Insurance companies have medical directors whose job is to balance health information with cost. Find out the name of this person, and send her all of your information. She may see the justification of your claim and step in to make a final decision sooner rather than later in order to cut down on the wasted time of her staff. Remember, most of the people you come into contact with aren't decision makers.

Going to the State Insurance Board

If the insurance company denies your appeal again, you have the option to go to your state's insurance board if there is one. Some states will give you the chance to have your claim reviewed by an external panel of experts. If so, the panel's decision is the final word in the case.

> **Code Red**
>
> If your insurance plan is self-funded by your company or organization, then your only option is to go through the legal system. You cannot go to an external review board. Keep in mind, though, that most self-funded plans are administered by insurance companies, so you may not even know that your plan is self-funded. Ask your benefits administrator about the details.

Forty-two states and the District of Columbia have independent review boards, and each state has its own laws regarding external review boards. Some states, for example, allow patients to sue their managed care plans for malpractice if a claim or treatment is denied.

Do not take the step of going to an external review board without first going through the internal appeal process, as some insurance regulations require the policy holder to work with the insurance carrier as much as possible.

Don't feel like a state independent review is a lost cause. The board is made up of physicians who specialize in the area of medicine under dispute. So the people you deal with now may be much more familiar with the treatment than the insurance company medical director you dealt with previously.

You can appeal any type of denial of benefits, although some state independent review boards impose restrictions on the type of provider, the nature of the procedure, or the dollar value of a disputed claim that they will review. And many states have time limits in which you must file your claim. For example, ERISA (the Employer Retirement Income Security Act), which applies to most insurance benefits obtained through a place of employment, requires claimants to file appeals within 180 days.

You are the person who is ultimately responsible for the bill, so not being able to pay it could end up being a real problem. Do all you can to get the charges paid, dropped, or reduced in order to make sure your credit doesn't suffer because of unpaid medical bills.

You do not need an attorney to file an appeal with the state. Just like your insurance contract, the appeal requirements are supposed to be written to be easily understood by people who have never been to law school.

Hiring a Lawyer

It may be hard to imagine how you would ever manage to hire a lawyer when you can't afford to pay your bills or perhaps pay for better health care, but when it comes to denied claims, it is sometimes necessary. The reality is that medical bills can quickly add up and sometimes you have to spend money to save money.

Code Red

After an accident, illness, or the identification of a medical condition, your insurance company cannot drop you from their plan under the federal HIPAA law. However, if you don't pay your bills, such as your premium or co-payments, your policy can be dropped regardless of your health condition. And, remember, it is more difficult to get insurance coverage if you lose it for more than 63 days at any given time.

If you do decide to meet with a lawyer, definitely find one who specializes in health insurance issues. The laws and regulations are so particular and change so frequently that it will pay off. And use your intuition (or find out through a friend or by reputation) to ask yourself if you have an honest lawyer so he will tell you if you truly have a case.

When you are one person fighting a large insurance company, it can feel like there is no way you will ever win, and we don't deny that fighting for your rights is a daunting task. But you do have rights, and remember that appeals of denied claims often succeed.

Bet You Didn't Know

The leading cause of personal bankruptcy in America is unpaid medical bills, according to a Harvard study.

The Least You Need to Know

- ◆ Ask your insurance company about its appeals process, and follow their rules to the letter, paying special attention to their deadlines.

- ◆ Get every piece of information in writing, and send all correspondence to the provider as well as the insurance company, so they will work with you, as well as each other, to resolve the matter.

- ◆ Find out the laws in your specific state regarding appeals and denied claims; be polite with the insurance company and providers, but let them know, too, that you understand your rights.

- ◆ Call your state insurance board with all of the information, including dates, in hand.

- ◆ Hire a lawyer only if the amount of the bill justifies the expense and the lawyer feels you have a reasonable chance of success.

Chapter 14

Pay the Bill On Your Own Time

In This Chapter

- ◆ Don't panic!
- ◆ Understanding the details of your bill
- ◆ The time and plan for negotiation
- ◆ Charity is not a bad word
- ◆ Work out some plan

It's scary enough to be sick—or have someone you love get sick—without having to worry about the bill. Going to the mailbox each day dreading a white envelope with your name on it may be, for you, more stressful than the actual illness. Staying healthy is one of the keys to happiness but so is not having to worry about money.

If health-care bills and lack of money are causing you stress right now, we want to say, "Relax, we can help." You're not alone, of course. Unfortunately, plenty of people have been in this situation and felt the way you feel. Our job is to help you come out of this situation in better health and able to sleep peacefully at night because you aren't worrying about your finances.

Doing the Legwork

First, you need to accept one fact: dealing successfully with medical bills, especially if they seem out of control, will take some legwork, including phone calls, letters, and negotiations. You must make sure both that your bill is correct and that you can create a plan that will allow you to eliminate as much of the bill as possible and be able to pay the rest without having too many sleepless nights.

Patients with insurance not only get all or part of their medical bills paid, but they also get another side benefit. Due to their power, insurance companies negotiate with doctors, hospitals, and other providers to get the best prices for services. So if a patient does have to spend some money out-of-pocket, she will get a discount on those bills.

The uninsured, however, do not have the benefit of PPO or network discounts—so doctors and hospitals will often bill you at the "list" price. But you don't necessarily have to pay those high prices. You can do what the insurance companies do—learn more about the system so that you can negotiate with power and thus lower your bills.

Itemize and Clarify

Whether your bill is from a hospital or a doctor, make sure you understand what you are being asked to pay for. Request a copy of the itemized bill, especially for inpatient hospital bills where multiple charges are billed. Doctors' bills are typically easier to understand than hospital and lab bills, although all of them may have codes and abbreviations in them.

If you have any questions about your bill, call the provider's billing office and ask for an explanation. They may need to talk to the doctor or other provider to clarify items in question.

Asking questions about the bill and explaining that you believe you aren't being properly charged may buy you a little time, too. For example, if the provider is asking that you pay the bill in 60 days, then they shouldn't demand payment until all questions are resolved and both parties—you and the provider—have agreed upon an amount. Make sure you ask to have the bill "pended" until all questions are resolved.

Bet You Didn't Know

Three entities are involved in your health-care bill. The first is you, the patient; second is the provider—a doctor, hospital, lab, clinic, pharmacy, medical equipment company, or other person or institution providing a service. Finally, there is the payer, which might be you, but could also be an insurance company, someone who is helping you, or another source of money, such as a charity.

Reading the Bill

Hospital bills are difficult to read because codes are used rather than spelling out the names of equipment, tests, and services. Unfortunately, this shorthand presents a number of problems for patients and those who pay the bills. First, because figuring out what the codes mean is difficult, you can't tell if you are being charged properly or not.

If codes are on your bill (and they will be), call the billing department, and ask them to translate what each one means. This is exactly what an insurance company would do if they were questioning the cost on a bill.

If you have partial insurance or are submitting the bill to any third party for any reason, you will receive an *EOB—Explanation Of Benefits*—from the company. This will tell you how much of the bill the third party will pay and therefore, how much of the bill you are responsible for.

def•i•ni•tion

EOB stands for Explanation of Benefits. This long and sometimes confusing form tells what products and procedures the insurance company will pay for and what you, the patient, are responsible for.

Also request a copy of your medical records so you can compare it to the billing records. You have every right to your records although the provider may legitimately bill a copying fee. And, in fact, you should always leave the hospital with, at the very least, your discharge summary, so you can use it for your payment records as well as your health records.

Watch for Billing Errors

Watch for accidental billing errors, such as these examples:

◆ Duplicate billing: Being charged twice (or more) for the same items, services, medicines, or supplies.

◆ OR time: If someone was waiting for you while you were in surgery, ask them what time you got out or if you went in late. If you don't have someone who knew the time, you can find out how long you were in the operating room by asking the anesthesiologist or your surgeon.

◆ Length of stay: It sounds too simple to be true, but double check the days listed on your bill. Be sure you aren't being charged for days you were not actually in the hospital. This is also important if you were being transferred from one unit to another (such as the intensive care unit) or if, as is sometimes the case, your doctor said you could leave the Intensive Care Unit, but no regular hospital bed was available, so you spent extra days in a more expensive unit. This is also true for transfers between other units, such as post-operative or surgical. Each unit has its own price.

◆ Changed or cancelled services: If your doctor ordered a test, such as X-rays or blood work, but it was changed or cancelled, it's possible you were mistakenly charged.

◆ Typing errors: Everyone makes simple mistakes, so it's not impossible that you will be charged, for example, $15.95 for one aspirin rather than $5.95 for one (and that is just about what you are charged for aspirin in a hospital). Remember, bills are prepared by nonclinical staff trying to read the hieroglyphics of a doctor. The staff person can't read your physician's writing any better than you can, so it is reasonable to assume that mistakes will be made. It's no one's fault; that person is doing the best he can.

Ask About Prices

Finally, remember that hospitals mark up the prices of every piece of equipment they buy. People who have no insurance are almost invariably asked to pay the more expensive "list price." Insurers get a discount, and people who negotiate ahead of time also may get a discount.

Patients and payers often get irritated because of the prices of hospital aspirin, for example. The aspirin costs less than a penny if you buy it in the drugstore, but in the hospital, it is $5.00 a tablet. Well, remember it costs money to administer an aspirin—making sure it is noted in the chart means someone is taking care of you.

Rather than getting angry about a five dollar aspirin, pay attention instead to the prices of higher-ticket items. If they're administering a drug that costs the hospital $5,000, do they need to mark it up to $25,000? That's the cost that will make or break your budget! We know about a young girl who had scoliosis. She had a titanium rod put into her back and was charged $96,000 for it. That was just the cost of the rod; the whole hospital stay was $163,000. So, the payer wanted to know what the hospital paid for the rod. What is reasonable and customary for the drug or equipment being dispensed?

If the hospital won't reveal the prices, then go online to a medical supplier and do a little digging (see Appendix B). How much are the drugs or equipment typically sold for? You can call or e-mail the suppliers for price comparisons, then call the hospital back and tell them what you've learned. Remember, you can do this before you go into surgery (as we discussed in Chapter 12), but you can do the same research afterward and use your knowledge to get your bill discounted.

You can also go online to find out what Medicare would pay for a bill. Go to www.cms.gov, which has a listing of Medicare services.

For Your Health

All patients should bring a pad, pencil, and plenty of questions to their important medical appointments. In fact, if necessary, take a person to your meetings and also let him listen in on phone calls if you are worried you won't understand what your doctor and other experts are saying. Don't let insecurity or fear cost you money—and, more important, your health.

If you had elective or non-emergency surgery, call around to local hospitals and ask what they charge for the type of surgery you had. Then, go back and negotiate with your hospital, giving them the sample prices you were quoted. This information will give you some bargaining power.

Negotiation

Negotiation is an art (lots of books have been written about it), but you need to know two things right away: first, you need information or knowledge to negotiate well. Second, you need certain skills—such as the ability to remain level-headed and the ability to listen. If you don't think you'll be able to stay calm, consider having someone else negotiate your bill for you.

Getting the Information

So, let's start with the information. Ask a lot of questions about your bill and medical records. If the person you are speaking with can't answer your questions, ask to speak to someone who can, or if she is especially helpful and nice, ask if she can research your questions and get back to you. The medical and bill information you are researching is not just something that belongs to the hospital but also something that belongs to you.

Negotiating Effectively

The next thing you need to negotiate well is effective people skills. For the most part, you want to speak calmly and politely. Certainly some patients believe that yelling, making threats, and being demanding will get them the changes they're looking for, but we find two problems with this approach.

First, it will add to your stress level, which isn't helpful. Second, behaving in a threatening manner often ends any negotiations. If the doctor or hospital employees do not respond well to being treated disrespectfully (and, really, why should they?), there is less chance of a successful negotiation. In other words, you might then be stuck with a large bill and no other options.

Code Red

Do not complain about poor service at the same time you're negotiating the bill. The right moment to complain about poor service is at the time service is rendered, or immediately thereafter, and directly to the provider or someone in the provider's office. Complaints at the time of billing (usually months after the fact) are seen for what they are—a blatant attempt to reduce the bill by smearing the provider.

At the same time, you don't need to beg, plead, or ask for pity. If you were sick and the doctor and hospital helped you, they deserve thanks and appreciation, not to mention money for their services. Even if you need to ask for financial help or charity care, keep your pride, and ask for what you need in a way that allows you to retain your dignity.

So when negotiating the details of your bill, always be polite and sound as professional as possible. Knowledge of billing and medical terms will help convince the people you are dealing with to take you seriously and treat you with respect. Show respect as well, and try to enlist the person on the other end as your friend and ally. She did not invent this crazy system, and she doesn't have as much at stake since she's dealing with someone else's money (yours). Try to understand her needs (sincere thanks, polite treatment, prompt payment) as well.

Bet You Didn't Know

You can authorize someone to negotiate on your behalf. To do this, write a letter stating that you have authorized the specific person to get all the information she needs (i.e., access to your medical and financial records) in order to negotiate the bill. The hospital cannot release any information it has about you without your authorization.

Try to talk to the same person each time you call, and be polite and friendly so the person wants to help you. Remember, the billing department gets lots of unpleasant calls every day, so they will be happy to help the person who appreciates the work they do.

Keep in mind that you are in a good bargaining position—you've already had the work done, so the hospital now needs payment but can't deny you the service!

Remember one more thing: chances are whomever you speak with in billing has no authority to stop the bill or make an adjustment beyond a very small percentage. You need to find a person with authority who can actually give you the discounts or changes you want. Feel free to ask whomever you speak with, "Who has the authority to make a final decision about my payment plan?"

There are as many different approaches to this as there are people. If the bill is big enough, it might even be worthwhile to retain a professional negotiator or medical billing advocate.

Talk to Your Doctor

If you have no idea how much certain items or procedures should cost and if you suspect you are being incorrectly charged, ask your doctor—and his office staff—to help you get the typical charges. Explain your financial situation, and ask them to go over the bill for you. Ask your physician to give you an estimate of how much he or she thinks the bill—or items on the bill—should cost.

To fully explain the situation, you may have to write a letter to your physician because she may not have the time to listen to your story on the phone.

For Your Health

The Internet is a mixed blessing when it comes to health information. You should definitely use its resources in trying to determine if the tests and care you received at the hospital match your diagnosis. However, do not use it to diagnose yourself. See Appendix B, Resources, for reliable websites to use when researching your bill.

Once you have that information, call the billing department of the hospital and share the numbers with them. Explain that you want to negotiate how much you will pay. If necessary, fax, mail, or e-mail them your physician's financial estimates on the costs.

If the person you speak with in the billing department isn't helpful, ask to speak to a manager. If he asks to get back to you, keep calling. It's better to be a pain-in-the-neck than to have your bill be too expensive for you to handle and end up going to a collection agency.

When dealing with the insurance company, the provider is your natural ally; after all, they want to get paid. They will usually comply with any reasonable request from the insurer for additional documentation or explanations of their services. If they won't, simply explain that you are unsure of what you owe until the insurer has adjudicated the claim.

Keep careful notes, including copies of the bills, medical records, any insurance information, dates, the name of the person you spoke with, and written summaries of the information you received.

As a last resort, you can also go to the State Regulatory Agency to lodge a complaint about your bill, but be sure you have some reasonable argument. If you don't, they won't intervene on your behalf. Send a copy of the letter to the hospital because they might be tempted to work with you before a state agency steps in to investigate.

Many providers do extend some degree of charity care and will accept whatever you can afford as payment in full. You may have to speak with the doctor in person or at least the head of the billing operation.

Code Red

Do not pay the bill until you receive information from an insurer (an EOB) and an itemization from the hospital as well as your medical records (if requested). If the hospital demands payment before you have all the information, explain that you do not believe you are being charged correctly. Send a detailed list of your questions. If you pay the full bill up front, it may then become your responsibility to pursue a refund from the provider, which can be time-consuming and frustrating.

In some states, hospitals may extend charity write-offs if you can prove your income is below specified levels (this will require copies of your tax return). They are often reimbursed for a certain percentage of these "free care" write-offs by the states. Doctors, on the other hand, are not.

Call Their Bluff

If, in your negotiation, all else seems to be failing, you might try heaving a big sigh and saying, "I guess you'll just have to send me to collection." As in, a collection agency, but this is exactly where you really don't want to end up!

The billing agent on the phone will not care. However, the supervisor and the provider will fight to keep your account out of the collection agency's hands because these agencies take a "cut" of 25 percent or more off the top of what they collect and they collect on only a small percentage of their cases. Be sure at this point that you are talking to someone who has authority. The billing supervisor might well be persuaded that a 20 percent discount in exchange for immediate payment doesn't look so bad after all.

Hospitals will often even help patients—or potential patients—apply for insurance coverage through state insurance or welfare programs in order to assure payment.

Every hospital sets its own charity-care policy. Some will expect a charity patient to pay part of his bill; others will pay the whole amount.

def•i•ni•tion

Charity care usually refers to financial assistance that is given to people who live within some percentage of the federal poverty level. You will have to explain your financial situation—and prove it with documentation—to the hospital, but the care you receive will not be different. In fact, no one will know about your financial situation unless you talk about it.

Most hospitals will not pay for non-medical expenses, such as in-room television use or telephone charges.

And when it comes to determining your eligibility, they will look at your income, your expenses, and your debt. So, if the hospital finds out that you have expensive car payments or other debt, they might advise you to sell some of your favorite toys or change some of your habits. You don't have to take their advice, but, remember, they don't have to negotiate with you, either.

Not Everyone Won't Offer to Wipe the Slate Clean

According to The Access Report published in 2003, 32 percent of hospitals will suggest that patients pay the full bill in installments, while only 12 percent will offer to discount the bill. Oddly, though, 13 percent of the hospitals will offer to waive the bill.

The statistics above explain why 46 percent of patients who took part in The Access Report said they had unpaid bills (which will happen if you are paying on installment) or were in debt to the facility where they received care. And those patients who had used a hospital ER, or outpatient department (OPD) were most likely—about 2 out of 3—to report being in debt to their facility.

> **Bet You Didn't Know**
>
> Staff offers of assistance made a difference; the more often staff offered to find out about financial assistance, the less likely that respondents reported being in debt to the facility.

Being in debt to a doctor, hospital, or clinic affects more than just the present. Access Advocacy Group found that about a fourth of all patients said they wouldn't go back to a professional facility if they had unpaid medical bills. Now, this is problematic for a few reasons. First, if someone is sick, this might mean he won't go to the closest facility or get help at all. Second, when a patient believes that money destroys the relationship between a doctor and patient, then there is no space for that relationship to continue. So a trusting and knowledgeable relationship doesn't develop.

Because of these problems (which end up being just as professionally distressing and expensive to hospitals as they are to patients) many hospitals now offer their patients information about their billing departments as well as the names and numbers of financial counselors who help patients with their medical bills.

Using a Professional Bill Auditor

It is legitimate to question a bill even after it is paid. In the case of a substantial bill (such as a hospital bill for more than $20,000) it may even be worthwhile to retain the services of a professional bill auditor. This person, who usually works for insurance companies and often has a background in nursing or some other clinical field, will go to the hospital, review the medical record, and compare it to the bill to make certain that you got what you paid for. In the event an error is found in the bill, the hospital is obligated to pay back any overcharges.

Code Red

Ignoring your medical bills is the worst thing you can do because your doctor(s), hospital, or lab can turn the bill over to a third-party collection agency. This information may then go on your credit report.

Even though you don't have the power of a Big Insurance Company behind you, that doesn't mean you can't get the prices that they get. Do your research. Find out what the insurance companies are paying for the same services you received. That information is proprietary and contractual but, once again, bill auditors find ways to get the numbers they need for their clients.

Work Out a Payment Plan and Stick to It

Having a large unpaid bill is scary, especially if you are someone who has always had enough money and paid bills in a timely way. Even though many of us are used to paying off mortgages and car loans, having other unpaid bills is difficult.

And this is right where many patients get into trouble because they assume that putting the bill on a credit card would be preferable to owing money to a hospital or doctor. This is not true. Just because your hospital or doctor accepts credit card payments doesn't mean you should use one. And you absolutely do not have to use a card, especially one with a high interest rate.

While certain horror stories are told about people losing their homes over unpaid medical bills, we can tell you a more hopeful and realistic anecdote. Back in 1987, a high school senior and her boyfriend got pregnant and decided to get married and have the baby. Without insurance, money—or an education—they made a life together. Twenty-five years later—both with educations and business and with four children—they made the last payment to the hospital for the birth of their first-born child. The hospital was so impressed that this couple had actually stuck to the payment plan that they called the couple to thank them.

The Least You Need to Know

◆ Your goal is to pay the bill in a way that allows you to not be stressed or overcharged.

◆ You need to get more information than just the bill that is sent to you, so make phone calls and write letters, if necessary.

◆ Negotiation is a skill; if you have trouble with it, you may want to ask someone to negotiate on your behalf.

◆ Charity care is nothing to be ashamed of; if you think you need it, talk to your hospital about that option.

◆ Ignoring a bill or bills is the worst thing you can do because an unpaid bill can be turned over to a collection agency, which will affect your credit; so arranging a payment plan on a large bill is better than no payment at all.

◆ Many hospitals will allow you to make even small payments for a long time because they would rather get some money than send you to collection.

Glossary

affiliation period The time an HMO may require an individual to wait after enrollment and before coverage begins. HMOs that require an affiliation period cannot exclude coverage of preexisting conditions. Premiums cannot be charged during HMO affiliation periods. *See also* HMO.

Alternative Trade Adjustment Assistance (ATAA) ATAA is a benefit for workers at least 50 years old who have obtained different, full-time employment within 26 weeks of the termination of adversely affected employment. These workers may receive 50 percent of the wage differential (up to $10,000) during their 2-year eligibility period. To be eligible for the ATAA program, workers may not earn more than $50,000 per year in their new employment. Also the firm where the workers worked must meet certain eligibility criteria.

benefit Something an employer offers as an advantage above and beyond salary.

break in coverage A period of time when an individual has no creditable health coverage. Government-subsidized health plans may require candidates to have three months of creditable coverage before enrolling in the health plan. Some candidates may have a possible break in coverage of up to 62 days. If the break in coverage is more than 62 days, then some plans can impose preexisting condition exclusions.

certificate of creditable coverage   A document provided by a health plan that lets a person prove he had coverage under that plan and usually provided automatically when a person leaves a health plan. Certificates can be obtained at other times as well. *See also* creditable coverage.

claim   A demand by an insured person for reimbursement (technically indemnification) for a loss under the insurance contract.

COBRA   Stands for the Consolidated Omnibus Budget Reconciliation Act, a federal law in effect since 1986. COBRA permits a person and his dependents to continue in the employer's group health plan after his job ends. If the employer has 20 or more employees, a person may be eligible for COBRA continuation coverage when he retires, quits, is fired, or works reduced hours. Continuation coverage also extends to surviving, divorced, or separated spouses, dependent children, and children who lose their dependent status under their parent's plan rules. One may choose to continue in the group health plan for a limited time and pay the full premium (including the share the employer used to pay on his behalf). COBRA continuation coverage generally lasts 18 months or 36 months for dependents in certain circumstances.

continuous coverage   Generally, health insurance coverage that is not interrupted by a break of 63 or more consecutive days. However, when an individual joins a fully insured small group health plan, coverage counts as continuous if it is not interrupted by a break of 90 days or more. Employer waiting periods and HMO affiliation periods do not count as gaps in health insurance coverage for the purpose of determining if coverage is continuous. *See also* affiliation period, creditable coverage, fully insured group health plan, HMO, small group health plan, waiting period.

conversion   One's right, when leaving a fully insured group health plan, to convert his policy to individual health insurance. Rules cover conversion policies and premium charges. *See also* COBRA, fully insured group health plan, and HMO.

co-payment   A specified dollar amount that the patient must pay to the physician or institution each time a service or visit is requested. Co-payments are usually required at the time of service and are set by the insurance company (typically an HMO or a PPO) as part of the policy.

creditable coverage   Health insurance coverage under any of the following: a group health plan, individual health insurance, Medicare, Medicaid, CHAMPUS (health coverage for military personnel, retirees, and dependents), the Federal Employees Health Benefits Program, Indian Health Service, the Peace Corps, state health insurance high-risk pool, as well as certain coverage under state programs, policy or contract including short-term health insurance issued to an eligible individual, or policy issued to bona fide association members. *See also* continuous coverage, group health plan, individual health insurance.

eligible individual   Each insurance or health plan can set its own regulations, subject to federal and state laws, regarding who is able to enroll in a plan. For example, with the HCTC, "eligible individuals must meet all HCTC eligibility requirements, such as having qualified health coverage, not having disqualifying coverage, not being imprisoned, and not being able to be claimed as a dependent on anyone's tax return."

enrollment period   The period during which employees and their dependents can sign up for coverage under an employer group health plan. Besides permitting workers to elect health benefits when first hired, many employers and group health insurers hold an annual enrollment period, during which all employees can enroll in or change their health coverage. *See also* group health plan, special enrollment period.

EOB   "Explanation of Benefits." An insurance industry acronym.

Family and Medical Leave Act (FMLA)   This federal law guarantees up to 12 weeks of job-protected leave for certain employees when they need to take time off due to serious illness, to have or adopt a child, or to care for another family member. When a person qualifies for leave under FMLA, he can continue coverage under his group health plan.

fully insured group health plan   Health insurance purchased by an employer from an insurance company. Fully insured health plans are regulated by states and the federal government. *See also* self-insured group health plans.

genetic information   Includes information about family history or genetic test results indicating a person's risk of developing a health condition. A health plan cannot consider (and therefore exclude coverage for) a preexisting condition about which a person has genetic information, unless that health condition has been diagnosed by a health professional.

group health plan   Health insurance (usually sponsored by an employer, union, or professional association) that covers at least two employees or the self-employed. *See also* fully insured group health plan, self-insured group health plan.

guaranteed issue   A requirement that health plans must permit any person to enroll regardless of his health status, age, gender, or other factors that might predict his use of health services. If a person is HIPAA eligible, insurance companies must offer him a choice of basic and standard individual health plans that are guaranteed issue. Plans that are guaranteed issue can turn one away for other reasons.

guaranteed renewability   A feature in most health plans that means coverage cannot be canceled because a person gets sick. HIPAA requires all health plans to be guaranteed renewable. Coverage can be canceled for other reasons unrelated to health status.

Health-Care Group of Arizona (HCGA)   A state-run program that offers group health coverage to small businesses with 50 or fewer employees, including the self-employed, and political subdivisions (state, counties, cities, towns, school districts, and agricultural districts) as long as employers and employees meet specified requirements. The HCG plan is a managed care plan.

health care provider   A person or professional organization (such as a hospital) licensed to render medical services. This includes physicians, nurses, dentists, and others. The "class" of provider (i.e., an approved list) is included in insurance agreements and contracts.

Health Coverage Tax Credit (HCTC)   The HCTC is a program that can help pay for nearly two-thirds of an eligible individual's health plan premiums. In general, in order to be eligible for the health coverage tax credit, one: (1) must be receiving Trade Readjustment Allowance benefits (TRA), (2) will receive TRA benefits once his unemployment benefits are exhausted, (3) is receiving benefits under the Alternative Trade Adjustment Assistance (ATAA) program, or (4) is 55 or older and receiving benefits from the Pension Benefit Guaranty Corporation (PBGC).

health insurance or health plan   This term means benefits consisting of medical care (provided directly or through insurance or reimbursement) under any hospital or medical service policy, plan contract, or HMO contract offered by a health insurance company or a group health plan. It does not mean coverage that is limited to accident or disability insurance, workers' compensation insurance, liability insurance (including automobile insurance) for medical expenses, or coverage for on-site medical clinics. Health insurance also does not mean coverage for limited dental or vision benefits to the extent these are provided under a separate policy.

Health Plan Administrator (HPA)   An entity that provides or pays the cost of medical care and can include an insurance company, insurance service, or insurance organization (including an HMO), licensed to engage in the business of insurance in a state and subject to state law that regulates insurance.

health plan policyholder   Typically this is the individual who subscribes to the health insurance benefit. The other individuals covered under the policy are the policyholder's dependents. The HCTC-eligible individual does not have to be the policyholder of a qualified plan.

health plan year   That calendar period during which a person's health plan coverage is in effect. Many group health plan years begin on January 1, while others begin in a different month.

health status   A person's medical condition, both physical and mental, claims experience, receipt of health care, medical history, genetic information, evidence of insurability (including conditions arising out of acts of domestic violence), and disability. *See also* genetic information.

high-risk pool   Subsidized health insurance pools organized by some states. High-risk pools offer health insurance to individuals who have been denied health insurance because of a medical condition or to individuals whose premiums are rated significantly higher than average due to health status or claims experience. High-risk pools can be a form of qualified health coverage for the HCTC if they are deemed state-qualified. To be qualified, the high-risk pool must provide coverage to all individuals guaranteed coverage through HIPAA, not impose any preexisting condition exclusions, meet certain requirements for premium rates and covered benefits, and be officially qualified by the state.

HIPAA   The Health Insurance Portability and Accountability Act is better known as Kassebaum-Kennedy, after the two senators who spearheaded the bill. Passed in 1996 to help people buy and keep health insurance, even when they have serious health conditions, the law sets a national floor for health insurance reforms. Since states can and have modified and expanded upon these provisions, consumers' protections vary from state to state.

HIPAA eligible   Status an individual attains once he has had 18 months of continuous creditable health coverage. To be HIPAA eligible, one also must have used up any COBRA continuation coverage, not be eligible for Medicare or Medicaid, not have other health insurance, and apply for individual health insurance within 63 days of losing his prior creditable coverage. One is also HIPAA eligible if his health plan was not renewed by an insurer who discontinued offering and renewing individual health benefit plans. When a person is buying individual health coverage, federal eligibility confers greater protections on him than he would otherwise have. *See also* COBRA, continuous coverage, creditable coverage.

health maintenance organization (HMO)   A kind of health insurance plan that limits coverage to care from doctors who work for or contract with the HMO. These doctors generally do not require deductibles, but often do charge a small fee, called a co-payment, for services, such as doctor visits or prescriptions. If a person is covered under an HMO, the HMO might require an affiliation period before coverage begins. *See also* affiliation period.

indemnity   Protection or security against damage or loss.

insurance   A contract in which on person (the insurer) agrees to guarantee another (the insured) against loss caused by specified and agreed-upon causes now or in the future in return for the present payment of a premium (or regular amount of money).

individual health insurance   Policies for people not connected to an employer group.

IRS Form 8885   *Health Coverage Tax Credit*   An individual eligible for the tax credit must complete and submit IRS Form 8885 with his federal tax return in order to claim the yearly HCTC for months he was eligible but did not receive the monthly HCTC. The instructions for IRS Form 8885 provide guidance as to who may claim the HCTC.

IRS Form 1099-H *Health Coverage Tax Credit (HCTC) Advance Payments* This form provides the amount of monthly HCTC and the months to which the HCTC Program paid a health plan on an individual's behalf during the calendar year.

large group health plan One with more than 50 eligible employees.

late enrollment Enrollment in a health plan at a time other than the regular or a special enrollment period. A late enrollee may be subject to a longer preexisting condition exclusion period. *See also* special enrollment period.

look back The maximum length of time, immediately prior to enrolling in a health plan, that can be examined for evidence of preexisting conditions. *See also* preexisting condition.

Managed Care Plans A kind of health insurance plan, like an HMO, that can limit coverage to health care provided by doctors or hospitals who work for or contract with them—also called network providers— and therefore may limit enrollment to those people who live within a particular coverage area. A managed care plan may require a person to get permission, a referral, from his family doctor before he gets care from a specialist in the network. Some managed care plans will cover care at a lower rate if a member goes to a non-network provider or gets specialty care without a referral. *See also* HMO.

Medicaid A program providing comprehensive health insurance coverage and other assistance to certain low-income American citizens. All states have Medicaid programs, though eligibility levels and covered benefits will vary.

medical necessity A determination that a treatment, test, or procedure is necessary to a person's health or to treat a diagnosed medical problem. Cosmetic procedures, for instance, are not covered under medical necessity provisions.

medical savings accounts (MSAs) These accounts allow persons to save money (often on a pretax basis) from their paychecks for health care expenses. These expenses can include deductible amounts, co-payments, uncovered medical expenses (glasses, dental care, prescription medications), or expenses above the policy limits.

modified community rating   A requirement applicable to HCG plans that requires that the rate for each policy not vary due to the health status of those who buy that health insurance. Premiums can vary based on age, gender, income, and by county, as well as by health plan option and family status.

monthly HCTC program   A payment plan through which the HCTC pays the 65 percent portion of an individual's eligible monthly health plan premium as it becomes due. Eligible individuals must register to receive the monthly credit by completing the HCTC Registration Form.

National Emergency Grant (NEG) Bridge/Gap-filler Funds   Also called temporary state-level assistance for the HCTC, these federal grants are available to states to assist eligible TAA/ATAA and PBGC recipients by paying 65 percent of their eligible health plan premiums while individuals are registering for the monthly HCTC. Once an individual receives his first invoice for the HCTC, he no longer receives NEG funds from the state. States apply to the Department of Labor for these grants, and then individuals apply to the state to receive the available funds.

nondiscrimination   A requirement that group health plans cannot discriminate against anyone based on his health status. Coverage under a group health plan cannot be denied or restricted, nor can anyone be charged a higher premium, based on one's health status. Group health plans can restrict coverage based on other factors (such as part-time employment) that are unrelated to health status. *See also* group health plan, health status.

nondiscriminatory premium   This term means that a health plan can not charge anyone a higher premium than another equally qualified customer. Complaints about how premiums are set should be referred to the state's Department of Insurance.

nongroup/individual health plan   Nongroup/individual health insurance is an individual policy for a single person or family. This coverage is usually provided under a contract purchased through an insurance company, agent, or broker. In order to have the HCTC cover this type of coverage, the nongroup/individual plan must have started at least 30 days before the person left the job that made him or her eligible for TAA, ATAA, or PBGC benefits.

Pension Benefit Guaranty Corporation (PBGC)   This federal government corporation, established by Title IV of the Employee Retirement Income Security Act of 1974 (ERISA), encourages the continuation and maintenance of defined benefit pension plans and provides timely and uninterrupted payment of pension benefits to participants and beneficiaries in plans covered by PBGC. It currently guarantees payment of basic pension benefits earned by American workers and retirees participating in private-sector defined benefit pension plans. The agency receives no funds from general tax revenues. Operations are financed largely by insurance premiums paid by companies that sponsor pension plans and by PBGC's investment returns.

preexisting condition   Any condition (either physical or mental) for which medical advice, diagnosis, care, or treatment was recommended or received within the 6-month period immediately preceding enrollment in a health plan. Pregnancy cannot be counted as a preexisting condition. Genetic information about one's likelihood of developing a disease or condition, without a diagnosis of that disease or condition, cannot be considered a preexisting condition. Newborns, newly adopted children, and children placed for adoption covered within 30 days cannot be subject to preexisting condition exclusions. Preexisting conditions may not be covered by insurance policies.

preexisting condition exclusion period   The time during which a health plan will not pay for covered care relating to a pre-existing condition. *See also* pre-existing condition.

premium   Amount of money paid at specified intervals to purchase insurance coverage.

reinsurance   When risk is transferred through a contract from one insurer to another, which then pays all the claims of the insured.

self-insured group health plans   Plans set up by employers who set aside funds to pay their employees' health claims. Because employers often hire insurance companies to run these plans, they may look like fully insured plans. Employers must disclose in benefits information whether an insurer is responsible for funding or for only administering the plan. If the insurer is only administering the plan, it is self-insured. Most self-insured plans are regulated by the U.S. Department of Labor.

small group health plans   Each state has different regulations about these numbers, but usually plans that cover at least 2 but not more than 50 eligible employees or plans with at least one (self-employed) individual but not more than 50 employees.

special enrollment period   A time, triggered by certain specific events, during which an individual and his dependents must be permitted to sign up for coverage under a group health plan. Employers and group health insurers must make such a period available to employees and their dependents when their family status changes or when their health insurance status changes. Special enrollment periods must last at least 30 days. Enrollment in a health plan during a special enrollment period is not considered late enrollment. *See also* late enrollment.

subrogation   To substitute one thing for another. In health insurance it refers to when an insurance company assumes a legal claim on behalf of its insured—for example, when an insurer submits a claim against a third party (such as a hospital) for indemnification (reimbursement) of the claim already paid by the insurer.

Supplemental Security Income (SSI)   This program provides cash benefits to certain very low income, disabled, and elderly individuals. When one qualifies for SSI, he generally also qualifies for Medicaid. In addition, Medicaid coverage often continues for a limited time if his income increases so that he no longer qualifies for SSI. *See also* Medicaid.

Temporary Assistance for Needy Families (TANF)   This program provides cash benefits to low income families with children. When someone qualifies for TANF, she generally also qualifies for Medicaid. In addition, Medicaid coverage often continues for a limited time or longer if she no longer qualifies for TANF. *See also* Medicaid.

waiting period   The time a person may be required to work for an employer before he is eligible for health benefits. Not all employers require waiting periods. Waiting periods do not count as gaps in health insurance for purposes of determining whether coverage is continuous. If an employer requires a waiting period, a preexisting condition exclusion period begins on the first day of the waiting period. *See also* preexisting condition exclusion period.

Appendix B

Resources

There is no getting around the hard truth: if you don't have health insurance, you'll need to do a lot of the telephone calling and information gathering that insurance companies do for their members. We designed this section of the book so that you have somewhere to go when you need information, medical supplies, or support in your quest to get quality health care without insurance.

Remember: keep a notebook and a pen with you at all times when you make phone calls or speak with someone about what you need. It's also a good idea to have a folder (that may end up becoming a large binder or box) in which to keep all your receipts and paperwork.

You will need this notebook and folder so you always know where your information is as you make more phone calls and gather more information. If you do get private insurance or apply for government assistance, you will be asked for numerous copies of all sorts of paperwork: health information, identification sources, and previous insurance records.

Also, keeping track of whom you speak with and when will help you get back in touch with the people who have previously assisted you. Developing a personal relationship with the individuals in a government agency, an insurance company, or a medical office may help you get what you need.

It's a lot of work, to be sure, but remember that even those who get insurance benefits have to make lots of phone calls and often have to fight their insurance companies for coverage rights. In other words, the legwork you are doing is going on all around the country.

Medical Supply Companies

You can use the companies listed here to get prices for equipment, such as wheelchairs and oxygen tanks. When you have prices, you can use this information as ammunition if you need to prove that an insurance company denied a claim or if a hospital or other provider overcharged you. You can also purchase what you need directly from these companies. They all ship across the country and have toll-free numbers as well as websites.

Medical Supplies and Equipment Company: Houston, Texas. Visit www.medical-supplies-equipment-company.com or call (toll-free) 1-877-706-4480.

Medical Supply Group: New York, NY. Go to www.medsupplyco.com or call 1-888-MED-8282.

Medical Supply Company: Deerfield Beach, FL. Go to www. medsupplylco.com or e-mail support@medsupplyco.com or call 1-877-706-480.

Online Home Medical Supply: Van Nuys, CA. Go to www. onlinehomemedical supply or contactus@onlinehomemedicalsupply. com or call 1-888-311-0666.

O.U.C. Medical, Inc.: Tampa, FL. Go to www.oucmedical.com or call 1-800-783-9321.

Also, look on eBay under "Health-care-Lab-Life-Science" for used medical equipment.

In the phonebook, look under medical equipment, health-care supplies, and home healthcare.

Organizations That Offer Support to the Uninsured

Access Project: Helps individuals find health care in their community. Go to www.accessproject.org.

National Health Policy Forum: Works to inform Congress and other politicians on insurance and other policies. Go to www.nhpf.org.

Kaiser Family Foundation: A nonprofit organization working to help individuals without insurance. Go to www.kff.org.

Physicians for a National Health Program: Advocacy group working to get insurance for all Americans. Go to www.pnhp.org.

Cover The Uninsured: Advocacy for a national insurance system. Go to covertheuninsured.org.

Government Agencies

For SCHIP (children's health programs) go to www.slc. edu/health-advocacy/index.php.

HIPAA: Go to www.hipaa.org

To find out if you're eligible for Medicare or Medicaid, go to Centers for Medicare & Medicaid Services at www.cms.gov or call 1-877-267-2323. You can also go to www.medicare.gov.

Insurance Information

To find out if an insurance company you are interested in is well-regarded, look at A.M. Best: go to www.ambest.com.

To find an American insurance company, look at the America's Health Insurance Plan website at www.ahip.org.

To learn more about your health insurance rights, go to The Agency for Health-care Research and Quality (part of the U.S. Department of Health and Human Services): www.ahrq.gov/consumer/hlthpln1.htm.

National Council for the Aging Benefits Check Up: This organization helps the elderly get the correct health insurance. Go to ss1. benefitscheckup.org.

The Georgetown University Health Policy Institute offers *A Consumer Guide for Getting and Keeping Health Insurance*, a guide that summarizes your protections in every state and the District of Columbia. You can see it at www.healthinsuranceinfo.net.

Mental Health Care

For the National Mental Health Information Center, go to www. mentalhealth.samhsa.gov or call 1-800-789-2647.

Vision Care

Vision Care: go to www.preventblindness.org.

Financial Aid for Eye Care: www.nei.nih.gov/health/financialaid.asp.

Further Reading

Brock, Fred. *Health Care on Less Thank You Think: The New York Times Guide to Getting Affordable Coverage*. New York, NY: Henry Holt & Co., Inc., 2006.

Farmer, Paul. *Pathologies of Power: Health, Human Rights, and The New War on the Poor*. Berkeley, Calif.: University of California Press, 2005.

Rowell, Jo Ann C. and Michelle A. Green. *Understanding Health Insurance: A Guide to Billing and Reimbursement*. Clifton Park, NY: CENGAGE Delmar Learning, 2005.

Index

Q-R

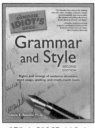
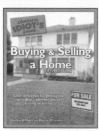
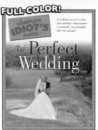
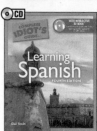
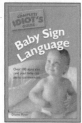
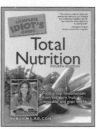
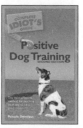
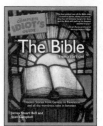
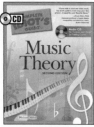
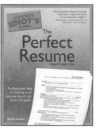
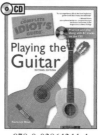
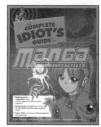
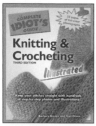
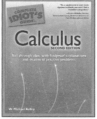
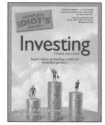